Kidney Disease Recipes for Newly Diagnosed

Easy solutions for a better living

By

Christine I. Stroud

Copyright © 2024 by Christine I. Stroud. All rights reserved.

All rights reserved. No part of this book may be reproduced in any form or by any electronic or mechanical means, including information storage and retrieval systems, without written permission from the author, except for the use of brief quotations in a book review.

This book is a work of non-fiction. All views and opinions expressed are those of the author. The author has made every effort to provide accurate information, but does not assume any responsibility for errors or omissions.

DISCLAIMER

The information contained herein is not intended to infringe, create or claim ownership of the app, software or tool of discussion. The app builder or product owner still holds full rights to their product as this guide is strictly for educational purpose. We do not claim any copyright or trademark ownership of any kind. Any views expressed are those of the Author, and do not necessarily reflect the views of any other person, organization or entity.

Table of Content

Introduction..8
Chapter 1..13
The Kidney Disease Diet...13
Chapter 2..19
Building Your Kidney-Friendly Pantry..19
Chapter 3..24
Breakfasts..24
    Low-Potassium Oatmeal with Blueberries...24
    Egg White Scramble with Spinach and Bell Peppers..............................25
    Chia Seed Pudding with Almond Milk and Berries.................................26
    Whole Wheat Toast with Avocado and Egg..27
    Apple Cinnamon Quinoa Porridge..28
    Coconut Yogurt Parfait with Low-Sodium Granola................................29
    Homemade Fruit Smoothie (Banana-Free)..30
    Baked Sweet Potato with Cinnamon and Walnuts..................................31
    Zucchini Fritters with Low-Sodium Feta..32
    Kale and Mushroom Omelette..33
    Almond Flour Pancakes with a Berry Compote......................................34
    Rice Pudding with Vanilla and Stevia..35
    Rice Cakes with Almond Butter and Apple Slices..................................36
    Cottage Cheese with Fresh Peaches and a Dash of Cinnamon................37
    Low-Sodium Breakfast Burrito with Turkey and Spinach........................38
Chapter 4..40
Lunches...40
    Grilled Chicken Salad with Olive Oil and Lemon....................................40
    Quinoa and Cucumber Salad with Greek Yogurt Dressing......................41
    Vegetable Soup (Low-Sodium)..42
    Lentil Salad with Cherry Tomatoes and Parsley.....................................43
    Rice and Bean Bowl with Roasted Veggies...45
    Tuna Salad with Cabbage and Light Mayo..46
    Stuffed Bell Peppers with Ground Turkey and Quinoa...........................47
    Chickpea and Spinach Stir Fry..48
    Egg Salad on Whole Grain Toast..49

Grilled Salmon with Steamed Broccoli and Brown Rice.................................. 50
Cauliflower Rice with Tofu and Peas.. 51
Zucchini Noodles with Avocado and Pesto... 52
Chicken and Sweet Potato Stew.. 54
Low-Sodium Hummus and Veggie Wrap.. 55
Toasted Veggie Sandwich with Sunflower Seed Butter.................................... 56

Chapter 5.. 58
Dinners... 58

Baked Lemon Herb Salmon with Roasted Asparagus...................................... 58
Chicken Stir-Fry with Bell Peppers and Zucchini.. 59
Grilled Turkey Burgers with Sautéed Spinach... 60
Quinoa-Stuffed Eggplant.. 61
Baked Cod with Garlic and Roasted Brussels Sprouts.................................... 63
Low-Sodium Beef Stir Fry with Snow Peas... 64
Chicken and Sweet Potato Mash.. 65
Vegetarian Lentil Stew.. 66
Turkey Meatballs with Zucchini Noodles.. 67
Roast Chicken with Carrots and Potatoes... 69
Grilled Shrimp with Cilantro-Lime Quinoa.. 70
Baked Tofu with Steamed Broccoli and Brown Rice....................................... 71
Stuffed Portobello Mushrooms with Quinoa and Spinach............................. 72
Cauliflower Crust Pizza with Low-Sodium Toppings..................................... 74
Eggplant Parmesan (Kidney-Friendly Version).. 75

Chapter 6.. 77
Desserts.. 77

Banana-Free Chocolate Avocado Mousse.. 77
Apple Crisp with Oats and Cinnamon... 78
Homemade Coconut Milk Popsicles.. 79
Low-Sodium Almond Butter Cookies.. 80
Berry Sorbet with a Touch of Lime.. 81
Chia Seed Pudding with Cacao and Almond Butter....................................... 82
Carrot Cake Energy Balls... 83
Baked Pears with Cinnamon and Walnuts.. 84
Gluten-Free Blueberry Muffins.. 86
Lemon Coconut Macaroons... 87
Rice Pudding with Stevia and Cinnamon.. 88

- Frozen Banana Bites with Dark Chocolate 90
- Baked Apples with Almond Stuffing 91
- Raspberry Sorbet with a Lemon Twist 92
- Homemade Apple Pie with a Nut Crust 93

Chapter 7 95
Snacks 95
- Carrot Sticks with Low-Sodium Hummus 95
- Baked Kale Chips with Olive Oil and Lemon 96
- Rice Cakes with Almond Butter and Cucumber 97
- Cucumber and Tomato Salad with Olive Oil 97
- Greek Yogurt with Berries and Chia Seeds 98
- Homemade Veggie Chips with Sweet Potato and Zucchini 99
- Air-Fried Sweet Potato Fries 100
- Cottage Cheese with Pineapple 101
- Almonds and Fresh Strawberries 102
- Apple Slices with Almond Butter 103
- Roasted Chickpeas with Paprika 104
- Peach and Mint Salad 105
- Low-Sodium Tuna with Cucumber Slices 105
- Rice and Apple Salad with Cinnamon 106
- Hard-Boiled Eggs with Fresh Herbs 107

Chapter 8 109
Meal Prep & Time-Saving Tips 109
- Day 1 113
- Day 2 113
- Day 3 113
- Day 4 114
- Day 5 114
- Day 6 114
- Day 7 114
- Day 8 115
- Day 9 115
- Day 10 115
- Day 11 116
- Day 12 116
- Day 13 116

Day 14.. 116
Day 15..117
Day 16..117
Day 17..117
Day 18..117
Day 19... 118
Day 20...118
Day 21.. 118
Day 22...118
Day 23...119
Day 24...119
Day 25... 119
Day 26...119
Day 27...120
Day 28.. 120
Day 29... 120
Day 30.. 120
Day 31..121
Day 32... 121
Day 33.. 121
Day 34.. 121
Day 35...122
Day 36...122
Day 37...122
Day 38.. 122
Day 39...123
Day 40... 123
Day 41..123
Day 42...123
Day 43...124
Day 44...124
Day 45...124
Day 46...124
Day 47..125
Day 48...125
Day 49...125

Day 50..125
Day 51..126
Day 52..126
Day 53..126
Day 54..126
Day 55..127
Day 56..127
Day 57..127
Day 58..127
Day 59..128
Day 60..128
Conclusion.. 129

Introduction

The information that James had been diagnosed with chronic kidney disease (CKD) came as a shock to him when it was initially revealed. James had never believed that something as basic as his food could have such a dramatic influence on his health. He was 52 years old, a successful project manager, and he had a family. Many people had heard of renal illness, but he never imagined that it would affect his life. He was one of those people. However, a regular checkup found that his kidney function was deteriorating, despite the fact that he did not exhibit any visible signs, such as excessive weariness or edema. The doctor's comments, despite the fact that they were not wholly shocking given the history of hypertension and diabetes in his family, seemed like a heavy weight weighing on his chest. The doctor's diagnosis was that your kidneys were not working as they should have been. It will be necessary for us to make certain adjustments to our lifestyle, most notably to your nutrition.

At first, James became disoriented. Although the concept of "dietary changes" was not new to him, he had heard it previously from health coaches, nutritionists, and even his wife; nonetheless, this time it seemed different to him. His kidneys were on the line. He had no option but to listen and act.

It wasn't simple, and it definitely wasn't fast. He was forced to reevaluate all he believed he understood about the relationship between diet and health. Over the next months, James steadily acclimated to his new lifestyle, and with a combination of meticulous food planning, professional advice, and a strong determination, he not only managed to stabilize his kidney function but also found himself feeling better than he had in years. He had more energy, his weight stabilized, and most significantly, he had recovered control of his life.

For James, the quest to greater health started in his kitchen.

When most people think of renal illness, they think of dialysis, doctors' visits, and an inexorable downward spiral. What James discovered through his trip is that this does not have to be the case. Kidney illness doesn't simply have to be controlled with medicine or dialysis; it may also be addressed by what you eat. The appropriate meal may be a great aid in managing the condition and ensuring that kidneys are given the best shot at keeping their function. It doesn't simply assist with controlling the symptoms—it may even reverse some of the harm done. And that revelation altered everything for him.

Kidney illness is a disorder that may take a toll on both the body and psyche. For individuals initially diagnosed, the emotional reaction is generally riddled with uncertainty. There are emotions of worry, irritation, and occasionally even rage. The first shock of diagnosis might leave someone asking, "How will I live with this? What do I need to change? What am I permitted to eat?" James' story mirrored the emotional rollercoaster many individuals go through following diagnosis. But along the process, he realized that, much as with any other chronic ailment, education, and understanding are crucial.

Kidney disease is a term that comprises a variety of disorders that impact kidney function. The kidneys, two bean-shaped organs in the lower back, perform a key function in sustaining human health. They filter waste and surplus fluids from the blood, control blood pressure, and create hormones that impact red blood cell synthesis and calcium absorption. When the kidneys get damaged and are unable to execute these critical jobs adequately, the body begins to retain waste materials and fluids, leading to different health concerns. Chronic kidney disease is frequently the consequence of long-term damage that builds over time.

Unfortunately, kidney disease is sometimes considered a "silent disease" since its symptoms might be minor or go undiagnosed until the problem has severely advanced. By the time many patients are identified, they may already be in the early stages of renal failure, when severe damage has already happened. The symptoms of kidney disease might vary, but they often include weariness, swelling in the feet, ankles, or legs, changes in urine, high blood pressure, and back or side discomfort. In certain situations, patients may feel nausea, vomiting, and trouble breathing.

The most prevalent causes of kidney illness include disorders such as high blood pressure, diabetes, and a family history of kidney difficulties. Both high blood pressure and diabetes damage the blood arteries in the kidneys, limiting their capacity to function normally. Risk factors include obesity, smoking, age (especially over 60), and a history of cardiovascular disease.

What many people don't understand, however, is that kidney disease may be slowed down, and in some instances even avoided, by early intervention, lifestyle modifications, and, critically, dietary improvements. This is where diet plays a vital role in treating renal disease.

Diet is one of the most effective weapons in reducing the course of renal disease and avoiding additional damage. When your kidneys are impaired, they can no longer effectively eliminate extra waste, water, and certain minerals (such as salt, potassium, and phosphorus) from the blood. As a consequence, these minerals may build in the body, leading to difficulties including fluid retention, high blood pressure, cardiac problems, and bone damage. By regulating your intake of these minerals, particularly via food, you may assist ease the burden off your kidneys and lessen their workload.

The thought that food might effect kidney health may be unexpected to some, but in truth, nutrition is a cornerstone of controlling the condition. Foods that are high in potassium, phosphorus, and salt might make the kidneys work harder, raising the risk of additional injury. For those with renal illness, some foods—like bananas, tomatoes, potatoes, processed meats, and dairy—need to be reduced or avoided totally. On the flip side, eating kidney-friendly foods such as whole grains, lean meats, veggies, fruits low in potassium, and healthy fats, may deliver necessary nutrients while maintaining kidney function.

The purpose of a kidney-friendly diet is not only about limitation, but also about making sensible choices that give the body with critical nutrients without overflowing the kidneys. It's about balance—understanding which foods may assist preserve health and which ones may cause damage. Through this information, persons with kidney illness may make choices that enable them to live a fuller life, despite their diagnosis.

James' story is a proof to the significance of food in controlling renal illness. After months of trial and error, visits with a renal expert, and working with a dietician, he came to grasp how the food he consumed affected his health. At first, he was overwhelmed by the limits. But eventually, he came to learn that he could still eat tasty meals while keeping his kidneys healthy. He found that his plates didn't have to be empty or bland—he could produce vivid, nutrient-dense meals that would fuel his body and support his kidney function. He began replacing out high-potassium items like tomatoes and potatoes with lower-potassium ones like cauliflower and bell peppers. He lowered his sodium consumption by using fresh herbs and spices instead of salt, and he learned to read food labels more carefully to avoid hidden sources of sodium and phosphorus.

With every meal that was meticulously prepared, James observed improvements—not only in his kidney function, but in his general health. He no longer felt exhausted, his blood pressure regulated, and he even shed a little of weight. His energy levels rose, and he found himself enjoying life again. His confidence rose as he learned more about the relationship between diet and renal function. This wasn't just about surviving renal illness; it was about flourishing.

For many individuals, a kidney disease diagnosis seems like the end of an era. It's easy to feel disheartened and overwhelmed by the work ahead. But as James' tale indicates, a kidney disease diagnosis may be the beginning of a new, healthier chapter in life. By taking control of the things you can control—like your diet—you can halt the advancement of the illness, feel better in the process, and empower yourself to take care of your health.

No one understands precisely why kidney disease occurs to one individual and not another. But what we do know is that early diagnosis and intervention may make a tremendous impact. By making smart dietary choices, avoiding the improper foods, and concentrating on nutritional meals, it's feasible to manage renal disease and continue living a meaningful life.

James now looks back on his adventure with a feeling of pride. What previously looked like a huge endeavor has become a part of his life's story, and he feels better for it. His kidneys may never return to full condition, but he knows he's doing all he can to safeguard them, and in doing so, he's living better than ever before. His experience is just one example of how a smart, proactive approach to kidney health may dramatically affect the trajectory of a diagnosis.

For everyone who has just been diagnosed with renal illness, there is hope. It's not just about survival; it's about flourishing. And it all starts with the choices you make—starting with what's on your plate.

Chapter 1

The Kidney Disease Diet

For most individuals, the kidneys are an afterthought—a pair of bean-shaped organs hidden down in the lower back, silently performing their work without any attention. However, for patients with renal illness, the kidneys become important to every area of life. Whether it's managing everyday tasks or making mindful selections about what to eat, knowing kidney function and its role in the body becomes vital.

The kidneys provide numerous key tasks that are necessary to health. They filter the blood, eliminating waste and excess fluids that are eventually expelled as urine. In addition to filtering out pollutants, they assist regulate blood pressure, manage the balance of electrolytes such as salt and potassium, and maintain the body's acid-base balance. The kidneys also generate hormones that play a critical role in red blood cell formation and calcium metabolism. Given the large and diverse role kidneys play, when they begin to fail or lose function, the effect on the body may be widespread and profound.

In the case of chronic kidney disease (CKD), this slow loss of kidney function may go unrecognized for years since symptoms frequently arise only after major damage has been done. As kidney disease worsens, the capacity of the kidneys to filter waste reduces, resulting to the accumulation of toxins in the blood, fluid retention, and an imbalance in vital minerals. This is where nutrition plays a vital element in reducing the advancement of the illness, preserving kidney function, and avoiding complications.

Diet is not merely a supplemental part of renal disease management—it is crucial. Making the appropriate dietary choices may make a huge impact in the course of kidney disease and can even help reduce some of the more unpleasant symptoms. Conversely, poor eating habits may accelerate kidney impairment and lead to further health difficulties, such as high blood pressure, cardiovascular disease, and bone disease.

For people who have just been diagnosed with kidney disease, the significance of food may seem daunting. What meals should you eat? What foods should you avoid? How can you make sense of the various limits put on your food without feeling deprived or discouraged? Understanding how diet effects kidney health is the first step in taking control of the illness and increasing your quality of life.

The kidneys' role is to maintain a delicate balance of fluids and electrolytes in the body. When kidney function is disrupted, it becomes more difficult for the kidneys to regulate this equilibrium. For example, they may struggle to eliminate excess sodium (salt), potassium, or phosphorus from the blood, generating harmful imbalances that may result in major issues including heart difficulties, bone disease, and high blood pressure. This is why dietary limitations are important to assist lessen the stress on the kidneys.

One of the first things patients with kidney illness learn is that regulating their intake of specific minerals is vital to sustaining kidney function. Sodium, potassium, phosphorus, and protein are the key nutrients that need to be carefully controlled, each for its own cause.

Sodium is one of the most hard minerals for individuals with renal disease to manage, partly because it's included in so many processed and packaged foods. Sodium causes the body to retain water, which may lead to high blood pressure, edema, and increased strain on the kidneys. When kidneys are operating effectively, they assist manage sodium levels, but when renal function diminishes, the body may struggle to expel excess sodium, leading to harmful fluid accumulation. Reducing salt consumption is an important dietary change for renal disease patients.

Potassium is another vital nutrient that requires careful management. Potassium helps control the heart's rhythm and is vital for muscular function. However, when kidney function is hindered, potassium may build up in the blood, which can lead to hyperkalemia—a condition that can trigger deadly heart rhythms and even cardiac arrest. For patients with renal illness, avoiding foods that are rich in potassium, such as bananas, oranges, tomatoes, and potatoes, is typically required.

Phosphorus is a mineral that is necessary for bone health and the production of teeth, but when the kidneys aren't working correctly, phosphorus may collect in the blood. High phosphorus levels may lead to bone disease, as the body leaches calcium from the bones to attempt to balance phosphorus levels. High-phosphorus foods, such dairy, nuts, and some meats, should be reduced in a kidney-friendly diet.

Protein, although vital for maintaining muscle growth and general health, may be troublesome for persons with renal disease since it creates waste products that the kidneys must filter. Consuming too much protein might put additional pressure on the kidneys. However, patients with renal illness still need to ingest enough protein to maintain their health, so maintaining the proper quantity is vital.

When it comes to foods that should be avoided, there are a few categories that are typically regarded off-limits for most individuals with renal disease, particularly as it advances. These meals are heavy in sodium, potassium, phosphorus, or protein and may impose extra stress on the kidneys.

Processed meals are frequently the greatest offenders when it comes to salt. Foods like canned soups, freezer dinners, fast food, and snack foods like chips and pretzels are often high with salt. In addition to producing fluid retention and high blood pressure, excessive salt consumption may further harm the kidneys.

High-potassium foods, including bananas, potatoes, tomatoes, oranges, and spinach, should be avoided or ingested in restricted quantities depending on the stage of renal disease. While potassium is a necessary component for the body, an excess of potassium may lead to life-threatening consequences, particularly if renal function is significantly reduced.

Foods rich in phosphorus, such as dairy products (milk, cheese, yogurt), nuts, and processed meats, should also be reduced. In persons with renal illness, phosphorus may build up in the blood, leading to calcification of the blood vessels and bones, increasing the risk of cardiovascular disease and bone fractures. Many processed foods include added phosphorus as well, commonly classified as "phosphates" or "phosphoric acid," which may be just as hazardous as naturally occurring phosphorus.

Excessive protein, especially from animal sources like red meat and fowl, may further stress the kidneys. While protein is vital for maintaining muscle growth, too much may generate an overflow of nitrogenous waste products that the kidneys must filter. This is why it's crucial for renal disease patients to carefully regulate their protein consumption, concentrating on high-quality, lean protein sources and ensuring that they do not ingest more than required.

Knowing which foods to avoid might seem difficult, but once you get the hang of it, it becomes easy to make educated decisions. To further help with this, reading food labels is a crucial skill for anybody controlling renal illness via nutrition. Food labels give vital information on the nutrient profile of the food, including the levels of sodium, potassium, and phosphorus it contains.

When reading food labels, always check the salt amount first. The American Heart Association advises that consumers take no more than 2,300 milligrams of salt per day, and preferably aim for 1,500 milligrams for optimal heart and kidney health. However, many packaged goods contain significantly more than this amount, particularly processed and canned foods. When feasible, pick fresh foods and avoid canned, packaged, or frozen meals that are high in salt.

Next, examine the potassium content of foods. Foods that are rich in potassium—typically 300 mg or more per serving—should be eaten with care. A potassium concentration chart may assist you discover which foods are healthy to consume and which are best avoided. If a product doesn't include potassium on the label, it's recommended to check a nutritional guide or chat with a nutritionist to verify its compatibility for your diet.

Phosphorus is typically present in foods that are processed or packaged, particularly those with added phosphates. This includes various soft drinks, processed meats, and snack items. Be on the watch for compounds like "phosphoric acid" or "diphosphates" on labels, since they signify that the food is rich in phosphorus.

When shopping for kidney-friendly meals, it's also crucial to concentrate on full, unprocessed foods like fresh fruits, vegetables, lean meats, and whole grains. By avoiding highly processed choices, you can reduce the quantity of salt, potassium, phosphorus, and other additives in your diet. Building a healthy shopping list that promotes fresh, nutrient-dense items can go a long way in helping manage renal disease.

Managing renal illness via nutrition may seem daunting at first, but with the correct information and tools, it becomes a powerful aspect of therapy. Understanding the function of the kidneys, how food effects kidney health, and the particular dietary limitations for renal illness are critical stages in the route to improved health. By making educated decisions and avoiding foods that strain the kidneys, it's possible to halt the course of the illness, feel better, and retain a good quality of life. With the appropriate attitude to eating, you can give your kidneys the support they need to flourish.

Chapter 2
Building Your Kidney-Friendly Pantry

When shifting to a kidney-friendly diet, one of the most critical tasks is setting up a pantry that corresponds with your health requirements. This adjustment might seem difficult at first, but with the appropriate components and tactics, it becomes not only doable but powerful. The idea is to create a setting where every thing promotes your well-being and every meal you cook feels like an investment in your health.

The key to constructing a kidney-friendly pantry is learning which foods are healthy and beneficial for your kidneys while also identifying the typical elements that might inhibit your success. For people treating renal illness, key minerals like salt, potassium, and phosphorus must be carefully regulated, so stocking your pantry with low-sodium, low-potassium, and low-phosphorus options is crucial. But this doesn't imply you have to sacrifice on taste or diversity. With a smart selection of products, your pantry may become a treasure trove of kidney-friendly alternatives that make cooking both pleasurable and gratifying.

Low-sodium spices and herbs are vital in a kidney-friendly pantry. Because salt is one of the first items to be decreased or removed in a kidney-friendly diet, these spices take center stage in providing flavor to meals. Spices like garlic powder (not garlic salt), onion powder, paprika, cumin, turmeric, and black pepper may offer depth and character to your recipes without the need for extra sodium. Fresh and dried herbs such as parsley, cilantro, oregano, thyme, rosemary, dill, and basil lend brightness and richness to dishes. Lemon juice, lime juice, and vinegar (such apple cider or balsamic) are good for increasing taste while being kidney-safe.

Healthy fats are another crucial component of a kidney-friendly pantry. Unsaturated fats, especially those from plant-based sources, are recommended over saturated and trans fats. Extra-virgin olive oil is a staple for its flexibility and heart-healthy properties. Avocado oil, flaxseed oil, and modest quantities of coconut oil are all wonderful alternatives. These fats may be used in dressings, for roasting vegetables, or as a basis for sautéing. Unsalted nuts and seeds, in moderation, may supply healthful fats, while patients with more severe renal disease may need to restrict their consumption based on their dietary requirements.

Grains and starches constitute the backbone of many kidney-friendly diets, delivering energy and adaptability. White rice, basmati rice, and jasmine rice are ideal alternatives for individuals wanting to reduce potassium and phosphorus, since they are naturally lower in these minerals compared to whole grains. Pasta (made from wheat or rice) is another terrific alternative, provided it's prepared without extra salt. For those who can take it, quinoa provides a nutrient-rich alternative with a slightly nutty taste. Cornmeal, polenta, and rice noodles are particularly worth adding for their diversity and versatility.

In addition to essentials, keeping kidney-friendly canned products may save time without sacrificing health. Look for low-sodium or no-salt-added versions of canned veggies including green beans, carrots, and maize.

Similarly, canned fruits packed in water or their own juice (not syrup) are wonderful for fast snacks or complements to meals. Low-sodium broths or stocks are another pantry necessity, providing as a basis for soups, stews, and sauces.

While stocking up on kidney-friendly foods, it's equally crucial to identify substances that should be avoided. High-sodium goods like table salt, bouillon cubes, flavor packets, soy sauce, and processed meals are among the first to disappear. Instead, look for low-sodium or salt-free options. For example, use coconut aminos or a low-sodium soy sauce replacement to replace standard soy sauce in recipes. Similarly, switch the standard salty broth with homemade or store-bought low-sodium alternatives.

Potassium-rich meals, while healthful for many, might be harmful for people with renal disease. Ingredients including tomato paste, tomato sauce, potatoes, sweet potatoes, and some canned beans frequently contain significant quantities of potassium. However, replacements may make these dishes kidney-friendly. For example, mashed cauliflower may substitute mashed potatoes, and roasted parsnips or turnips can stand in for potatoes in many meals. When it comes to beans, canned choices like black beans or chickpeas should be well washed to lower potassium levels, and even then, used in moderation.

Phosphorus additives are another hidden risk in many processed meals. These additives are typically found in deli meats, processed cheeses, baked items, and drinks. Look for ingredient labels that feature terms with "phos," such as "phosphoric acid" or "calcium phosphate," and avoid these items.

Instead, use fresh or frozen meats, natural cheeses, and entire, unadulterated meals wherever feasible.

One of the greatest ways to set yourself up for success with a kidney-friendly diet is to arrange your kitchen in a manner that fosters simplicity and efficiency. Start by cleaning your pantry and eliminating products that don't correspond with your nutritional objectives. This includes taking away any high-sodium sauces, potassium-rich canned products, or processed snacks. Once these goods are out of sight, replace them with kidney-friendly alternatives so that every shelf symbolizes your devotion to health.

Group comparable things together for easier access. Store all your low-sodium spices and herbs in one spot, preferably near your cooking area, so you can get them easily when making meals. Place healthy oils, vinegars, and other liquid seasonings together to ease your meal prep process. For dry products like rice, pasta, and canned foods, use transparent, labeled containers to readily recognize what you have and when it needs refilling.

Invest in a few kitchen gadgets that may make preparing kidney-friendly dishes more straightforward. A rice cooker may facilitate the preparation of low-potassium grains, while a blender or food processor can be essential for producing homemade sauces, dressings, and low-sodium soups. A spiralizer may let you produce kidney-friendly vegetable noodles from zucchini or carrots, delivering a pleasant alternative to conventional spaghetti.

In the refrigerator, designate an area for kidney-friendly mainstays like fresh fruits and vegetables that are lower in potassium, such as apples, berries, cabbage, and cucumbers. Store perishable foods like low-sodium cheese, unsalted butter, and eggs in easy-to-reach areas to promote their usage in meal preparation. Having a kidney-conscious meal plan displayed on the fridge will also help keep you on track and minimize the guessing when it's time to prepare.

Freezer space may be utilized wisely to store pre-prepared meals and supplies for rapid access on busy days. Portioning out cooked rice, grilled chicken, or chopped veggies into separate portions makes it simple to construct a kidney-friendly dinner in minutes. Freezing herbs like parsley, cilantro, and dill in olive oil cubes is another fantastic technique to preserve fresh tastes for later use.

A kidney-friendly pantry is more than simply a collection of products; it's a statement of your devotion to health and well-being. By stocking up on the correct ingredients, eliminating hazardous ones, and arranging your kitchen to facilitate ease of cooking, you create an atmosphere that supports success. Every meal you create from this place becomes a chance to take charge of your health, one kidney-friendly option at a time. With a well-prepared pantry, the route to improved living via food seems less like a task and more like a pleasant trip.

Chapter 3
Breakfasts

Low-Potassium Oatmeal with Blueberries

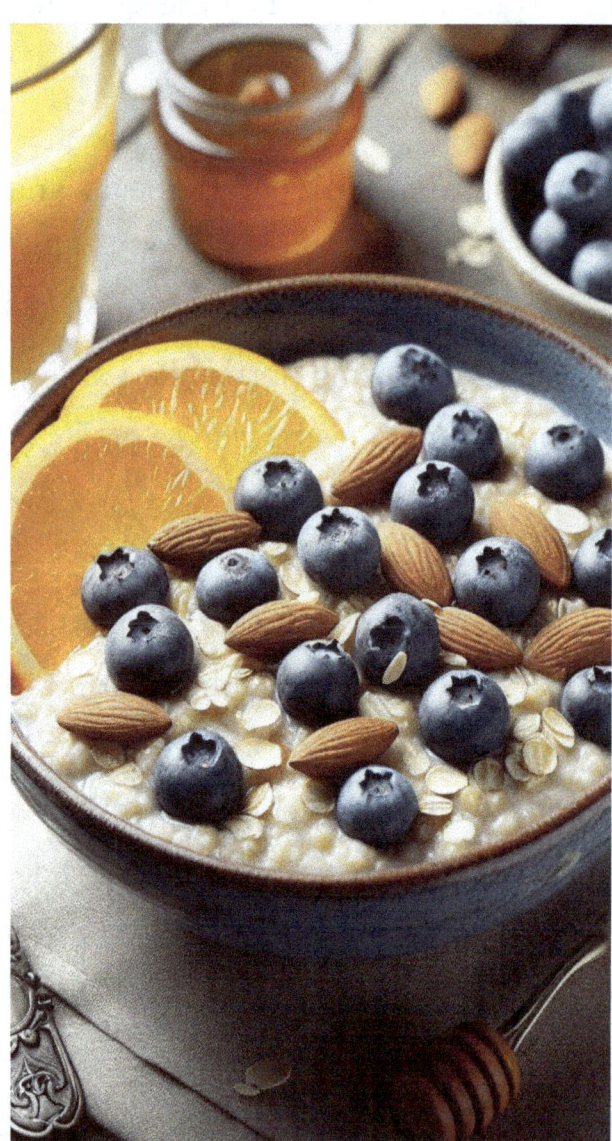

Prep Time: 5 minutes
Cooking Time: 10 minutes

Serves: 1

Ingredients:

- ½ cup old-fashioned rolled oats
- 1 cup unsweetened almond milk
- ¼ cup fresh or frozen blueberries
- 1 tablespoon chia seeds
- 1 teaspoon honey or maple syrup (optional)
- Dash of cinnamon (optional)

Instructions:

1. In a small saucepan, combine oats and almond milk.
2. Bring to a boil, then reduce heat and simmer for about 5-7 minutes, stirring occasionally until oats are tender.
3. Remove from heat, stir in chia seeds and honey or syrup if desired.
4. Top with blueberries and a sprinkle of cinnamon.
5. Serve warm.

Nutritional Information (per serving):

- Calories: 220
- Protein: 5g
- Carbs: 35g
- Fiber: 6g
- Potassium: 100mg
- Sodium: 50mg

Tip: For a creamier texture, add a splash more almond milk while cooking the oats.

Egg White Scramble with Spinach and Bell Peppers

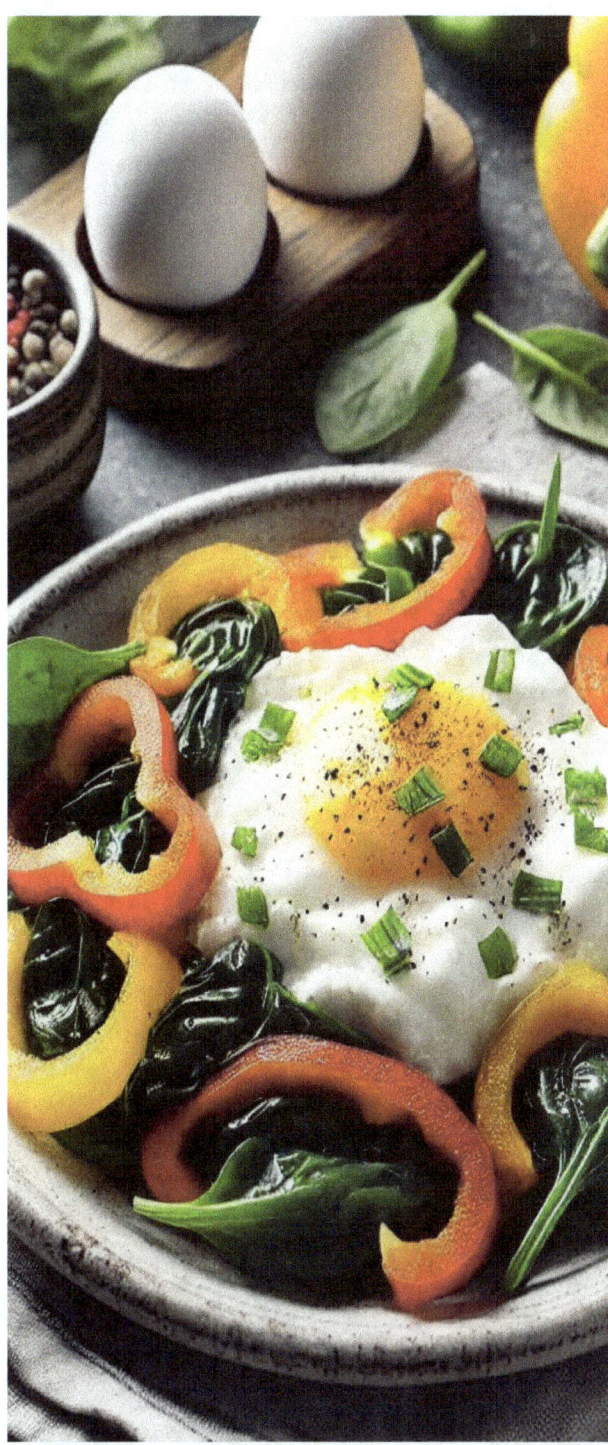

Prep Time: 5 minutes
Cooking Time: 5 minutes

Serves: 1

Ingredients:

- 3 egg whites
- 1 cup fresh spinach
- ½ bell pepper, diced
- 1 teaspoon olive oil
- Salt and pepper to taste (use salt substitute if necessary)

Instructions:

1. Heat olive oil in a non-stick skillet over medium heat.
2. Add diced bell pepper and spinach to the skillet and sauté until the spinach wilts and the peppers soften (about 2-3 minutes).
3. Add egg whites to the skillet and cook, stirring gently, until the eggs are fully cooked (about 2-3 minutes).
4. Season with salt and pepper (or salt substitute), and serve immediately.

Nutritional Information (per serving):

- Calories: 140
- Protein: 13g
- Carbs: 8g
- Fiber: 2g
- Potassium: 300mg
- Sodium: 60mg

Tip: For added flavor, try sprinkling a little ground turmeric or paprika into the eggs before scrambling.

Chia Seed Pudding with Almond Milk and Berries

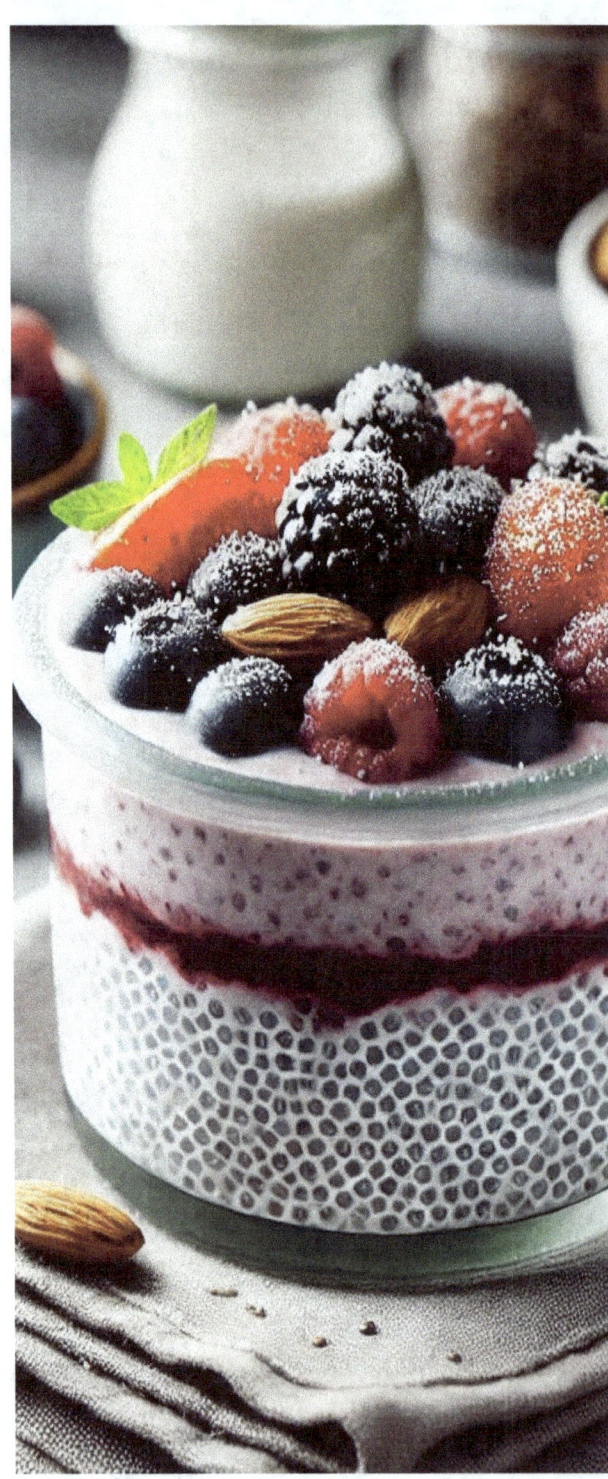

Prep Time: 5 minutes
Refrigeration Time: 4 hours (or overnight)
Serves: 1
Ingredients:

- 3 tablespoons chia seeds
- 1 cup unsweetened almond milk
- 1 teaspoon vanilla extract
- ½ cup mixed berries (strawberries, blueberries, raspberries)
- 1 teaspoon honey or maple syrup (optional)

Instructions:

1. In a bowl, combine chia seeds, almond milk, and vanilla extract.
2. Stir well to combine, then refrigerate for at least 4 hours or overnight.
3. Before serving, top with mixed berries and drizzle with honey or syrup if desired.

Nutritional Information (per serving):

- Calories: 220
- Protein: 6g
- Carbs: 16g
- Fiber: 10g
- Potassium: 150mg
- Sodium: 35mg

Tip: For a creamier pudding, blend the almond milk and chia seeds before refrigerating.

Whole Wheat Toast with Avocado and Egg

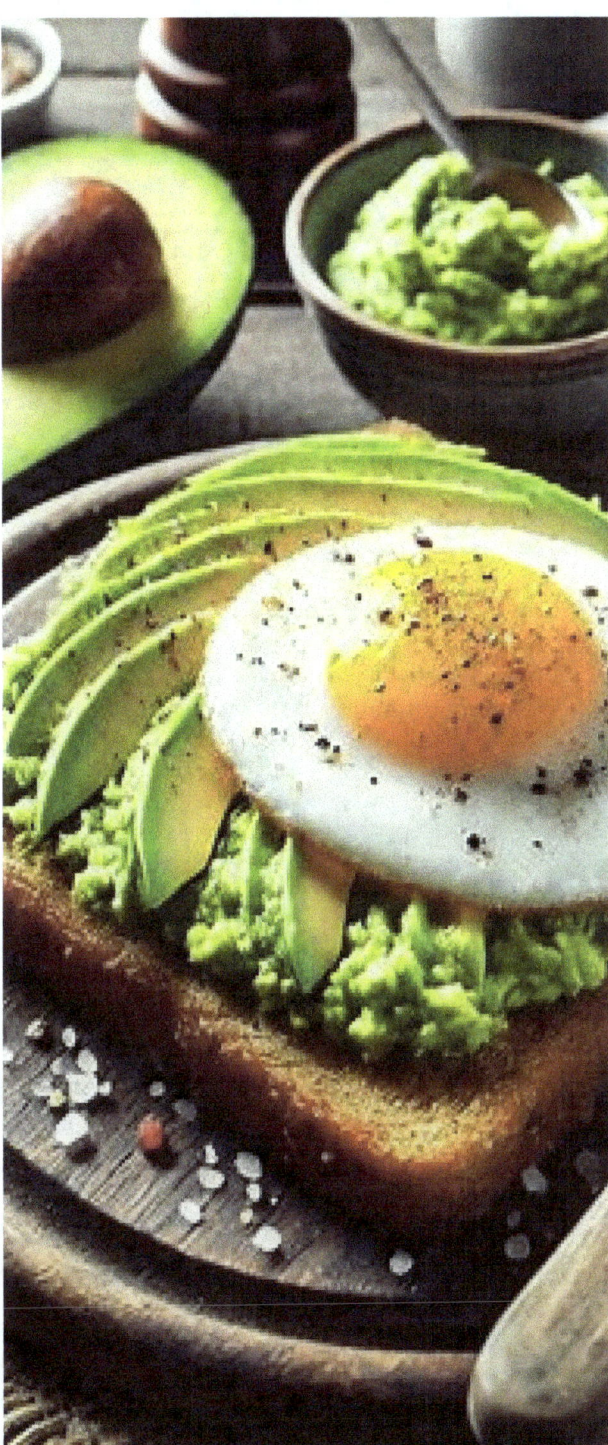

Prep Time: 5 minutes
Cooking Time: 5 minutes
Serves: 1
Ingredients:

- 1 slice whole wheat bread
- ¼ avocado, mashed
- 1 large egg
- Salt and pepper to taste (use salt substitute if necessary)

Instructions:

1. Toast the slice of whole wheat bread.
2. While the bread is toasting, cook the egg to your liking (scrambled, fried, or poached).
3. Spread the mashed avocado over the toast.
4. Place the cooked egg on top of the avocado toast, and season with salt and pepper to taste.

Nutritional Information (per serving):

- Calories: 280
- Protein: 13g
- Carbs: 24g
- Fiber: 6g
- Potassium: 400mg
- Sodium: 120mg

Tip: To add a bit of spice, sprinkle a pinch of red pepper flakes on top.

Apple Cinnamon Quinoa Porridge

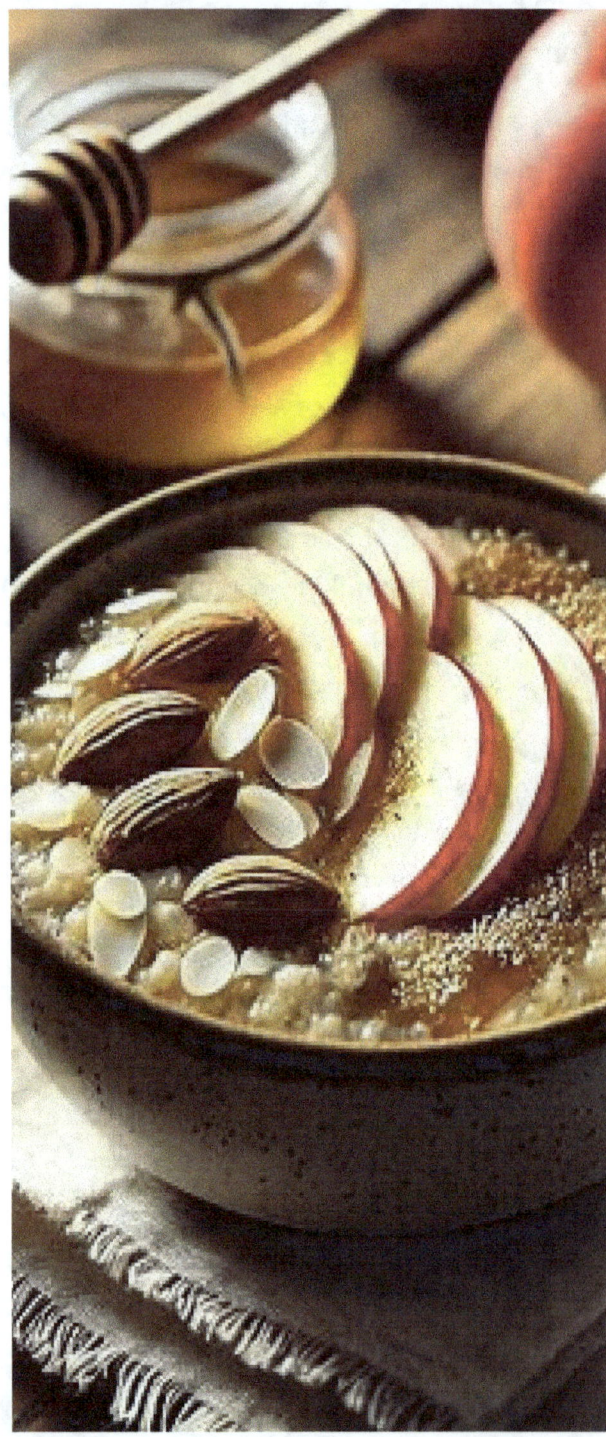

Prep Time: 5 minutes
Cooking Time: 15 minutes

Serves: 1

Ingredients:

- ½ cup quinoa
- 1 cup unsweetened almond milk
- 1 small apple, diced
- 1 teaspoon cinnamon
- 1 teaspoon honey or maple syrup (optional)

Instructions:

1. Rinse quinoa under cold water.
2. In a saucepan, bring quinoa and almond milk to a boil.
3. Reduce heat and simmer for 10-15 minutes, until the quinoa is cooked and the liquid is absorbed.
4. Stir in diced apples, cinnamon, and sweetener if using.
5. Serve warm.

Nutritional Information (per serving):

- Calories: 250
- Protein: 7g
- Carbs: 40g
- Fiber: 6g
- Potassium: 150mg
- Sodium: 40mg

Tip: If you prefer a creamier texture, blend the cooked quinoa mixture for a smoother porridge.

Coconut Yogurt Parfait with Low-Sodium Granola

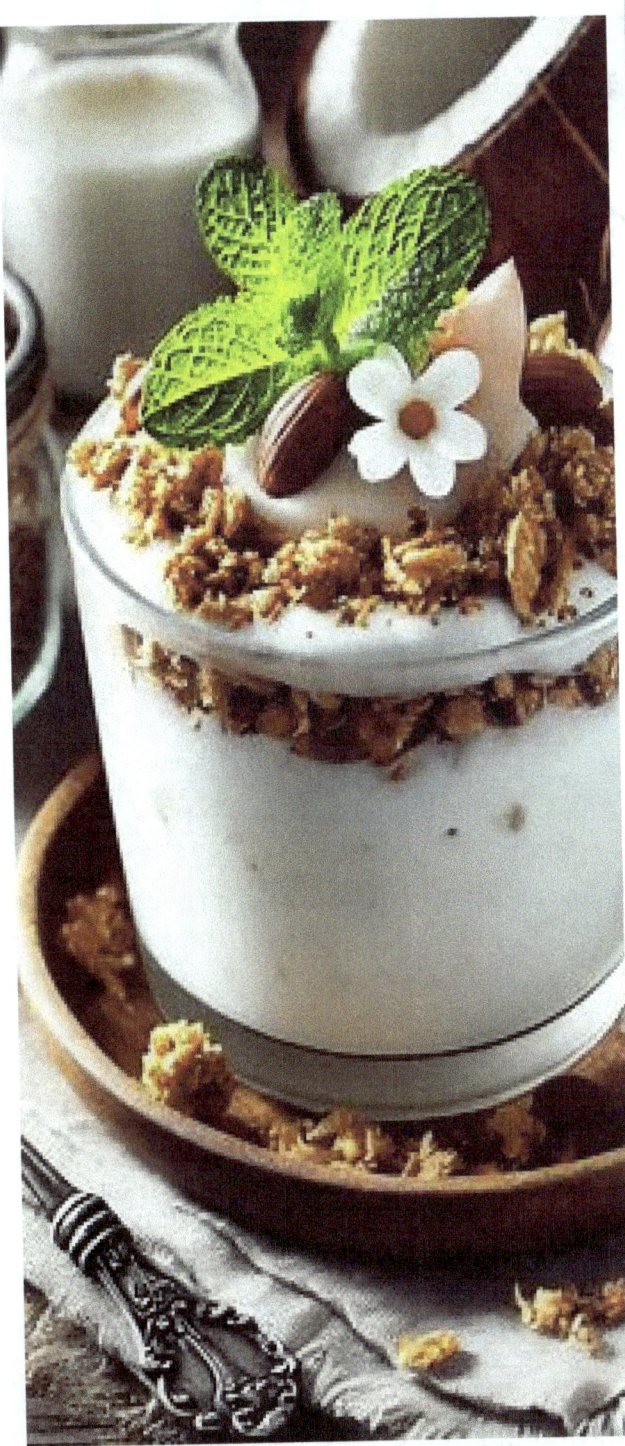

Prep Time: 5 minutes
Cooking Time: 0 minutes
Serves: 1
Ingredients:

- 1 cup unsweetened coconut yogurt
- ¼ cup low-sodium granola
- ¼ cup mixed berries (blueberries, raspberries, strawberries)
- 1 teaspoon chia seeds

Instructions:

1. In a glass or bowl, layer coconut yogurt, granola, and mixed berries.
2. Top with chia seeds.
3. Serve immediately.

Nutritional Information (per serving):

- Calories: 290
- Protein: 6g
- Carbs: 30g
- Fiber: 8g
- Potassium: 250mg
- Sodium: 55mg

Tip: For added crunch, toast the granola lightly in a dry pan before layering.

Homemade Fruit Smoothie (Banana-Free)

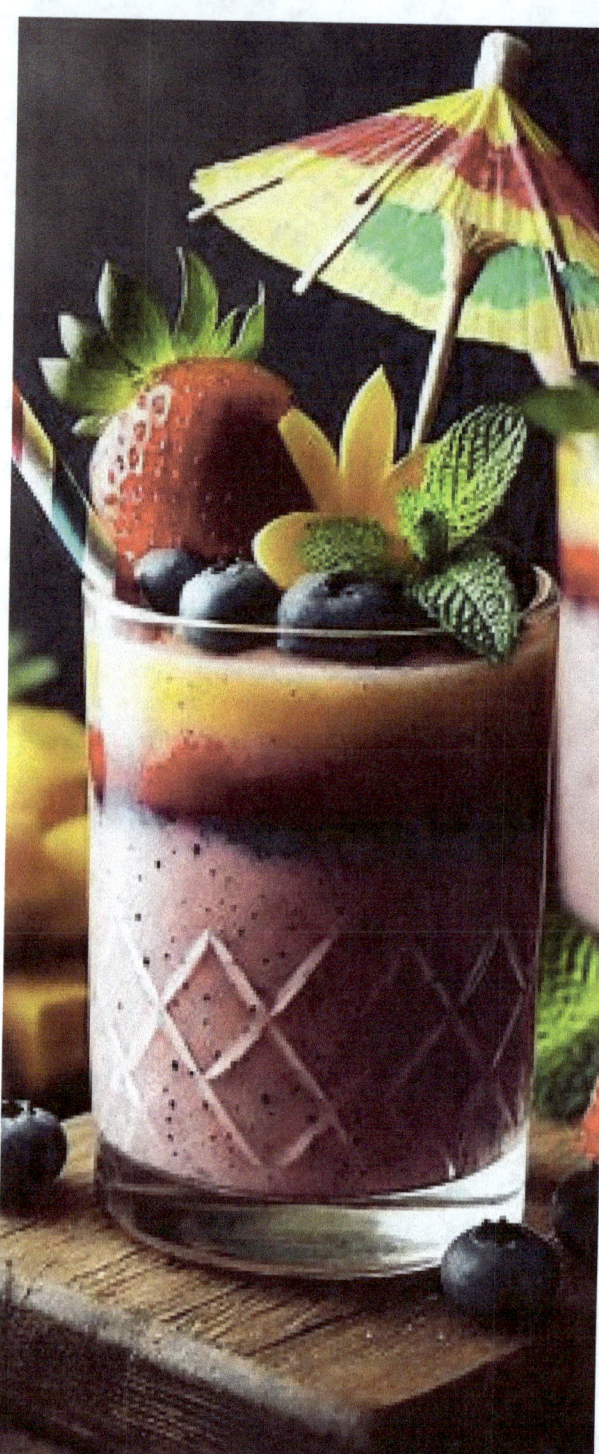

Prep Time: 5 minutes
Cooking Time: 0 minutes
Serves: 1
Ingredients:

- ½ cup frozen berries
- ¼ cup unsweetened almond milk
- ¼ cup coconut water
- 1 tablespoon ground flaxseeds
- ½ tablespoon honey or maple syrup (optional)

Instructions:

1. Combine all ingredients in a blender.
2. Blend until smooth.
3. Pour into a glass and serve immediately.

Nutritional Information (per serving):

- Calories: 150
- Protein: 3g
- Carbs: 20g
- Fiber: 7g
- Potassium: 130mg
- Sodium: 20mg

Tip: Use a variety of frozen fruits like strawberries, blueberries, and peaches for different flavors.

Baked Sweet Potato with Cinnamon and Walnuts

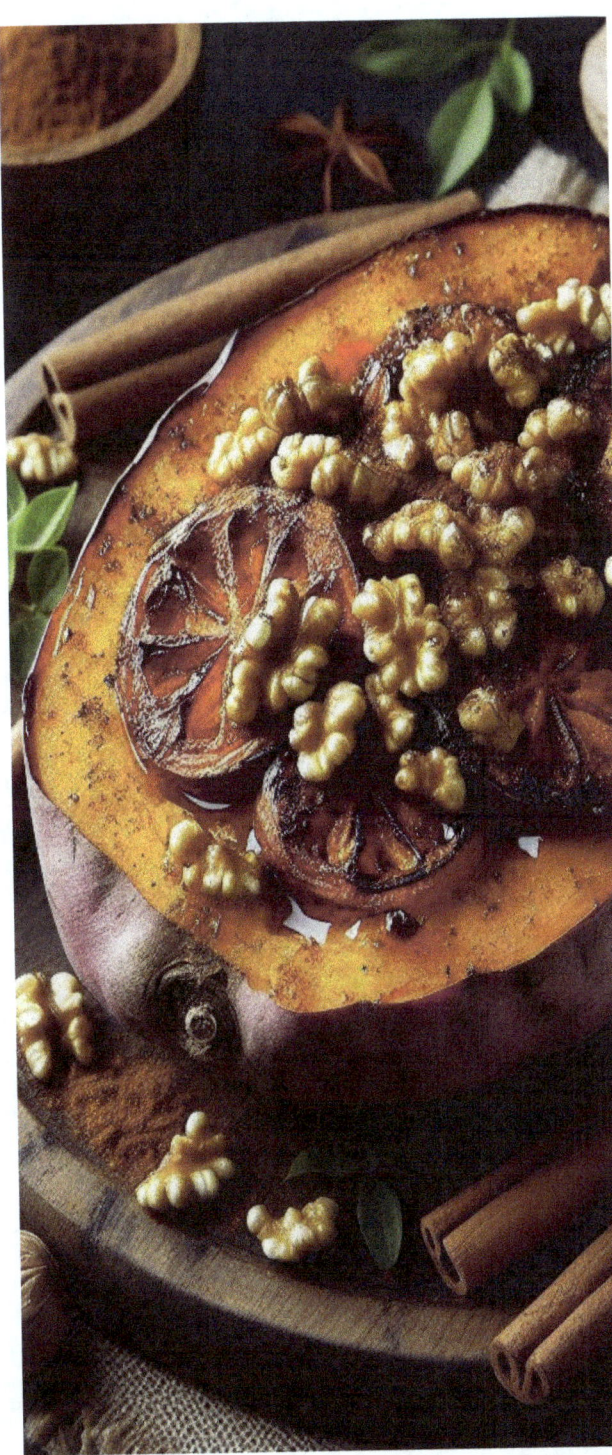

Prep Time: 5 minutes

Cooking Time: 40 minutes

Serves: 1

Ingredients:

- 1 medium sweet potato
- 1 teaspoon cinnamon
- 1 tablespoon chopped walnuts
- 1 teaspoon honey (optional)

Instructions:

1. Preheat oven to 400°F (200°C).
2. Pierce the sweet potato with a fork and bake for 40 minutes, or until soft.
3. Once cooked, slice open and fluff with a fork.
4. Top with cinnamon, walnuts, and honey if desired.

Nutritional Information (per serving):

- Calories: 220
- Protein: 3g
- Carbs: 48g
- Fiber: 6g
- Potassium: 400mg
- Sodium: 30mg

Tip: For a creamier texture, add a dollop of plain Greek yogurt.

Zucchini Fritters with Low-Sodium Feta

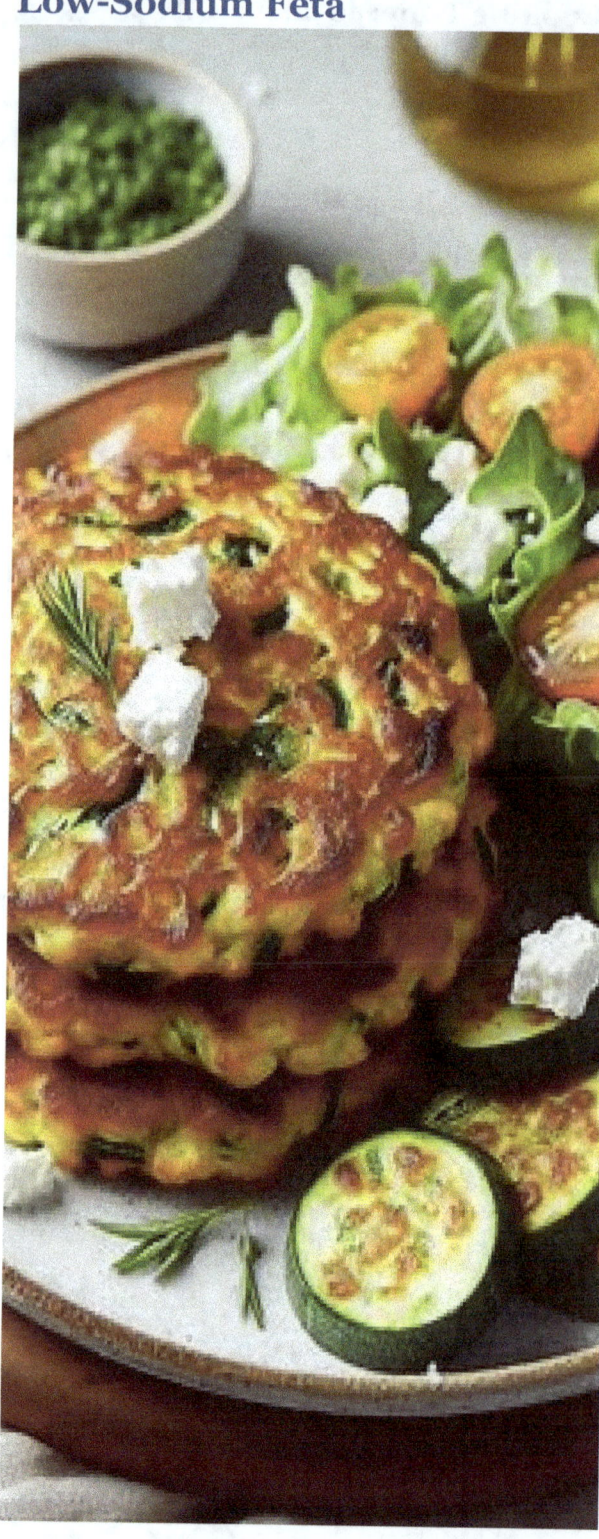

Serves: 2

Ingredients:

- 2 medium zucchinis, grated
- 1 large egg
- ¼ cup low-sodium feta cheese, crumbled
- ¼ cup whole wheat flour
- 1 teaspoon dried oregano
- Salt and pepper to taste (use salt substitute if necessary)
- 1 tablespoon olive oil (for frying)

Instructions:

1. Grate the zucchinis and squeeze out excess moisture using a clean kitchen towel or paper towel.
2. In a large bowl, combine the grated zucchini, egg, feta, whole wheat flour, oregano, and a pinch of salt and pepper.
3. Heat olive oil in a non-stick skillet over medium heat.
4. Spoon heaping tablespoons of the zucchini mixture into the skillet, pressing down gently to form patties.
5. Cook for 3-4 minutes on each side, or until golden brown.
6. Serve warm.

Nutritional Information (per serving):

- Calories: 150
- Protein: 8g
- Carbs: 12g
- Fiber: 3g
- Potassium: 250mg
- Sodium: 210mg

Tip: For an extra burst of flavor, add fresh herbs like parsley or dill to the fritter mix.

Prep Time: 10 minutes
Cooking Time: 15 minutes

Kale and Mushroom Omelette

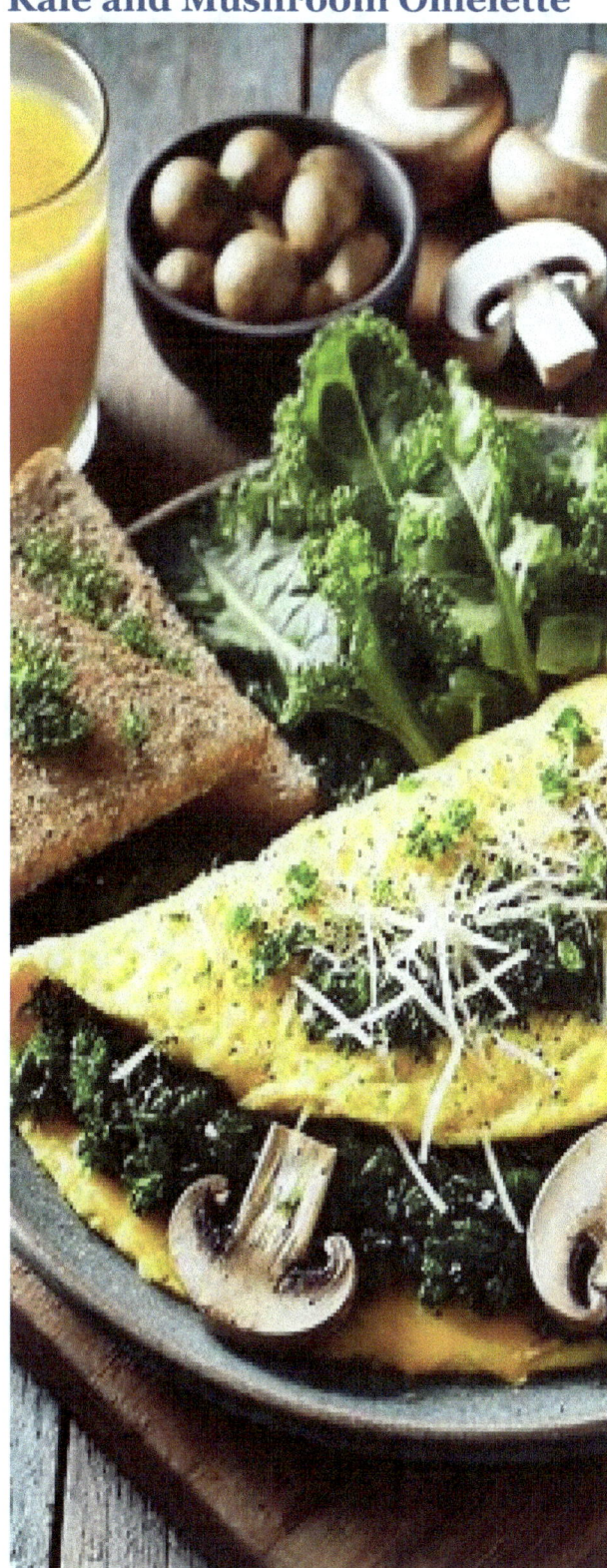

Prep Time: 5 minutes
Cooking Time: 5 minutes
Serves: 1
Ingredients:

- 2 large eggs
- 1/4 cup fresh kale, chopped
- 1/4 cup mushrooms, sliced
- 1 teaspoon olive oil
- Salt and pepper to taste (use salt substitute if necessary)

Instructions:

1. In a small bowl, whisk the eggs with a pinch of salt and pepper.
2. Heat olive oil in a non-stick skillet over medium heat.
3. Add the sliced mushrooms and cook for 2-3 minutes until softened.
4. Add the chopped kale and cook for an additional 1-2 minutes, until wilted.
5. Pour the beaten eggs into the skillet, ensuring they cover the vegetables.
6. Cook for 2-3 minutes, then fold the omelet in half and serve.

Nutritional Information (per serving):

- Calories: 250
- Protein: 14g
- Carbs: 7g
- Fiber: 2g
- Potassium: 350mg
- Sodium: 180mg

Tip: For a creamier omelet, add a tablespoon of unsweetened almond milk to the beaten eggs before cooking.

Almond Flour Pancakes with a Berry Compote

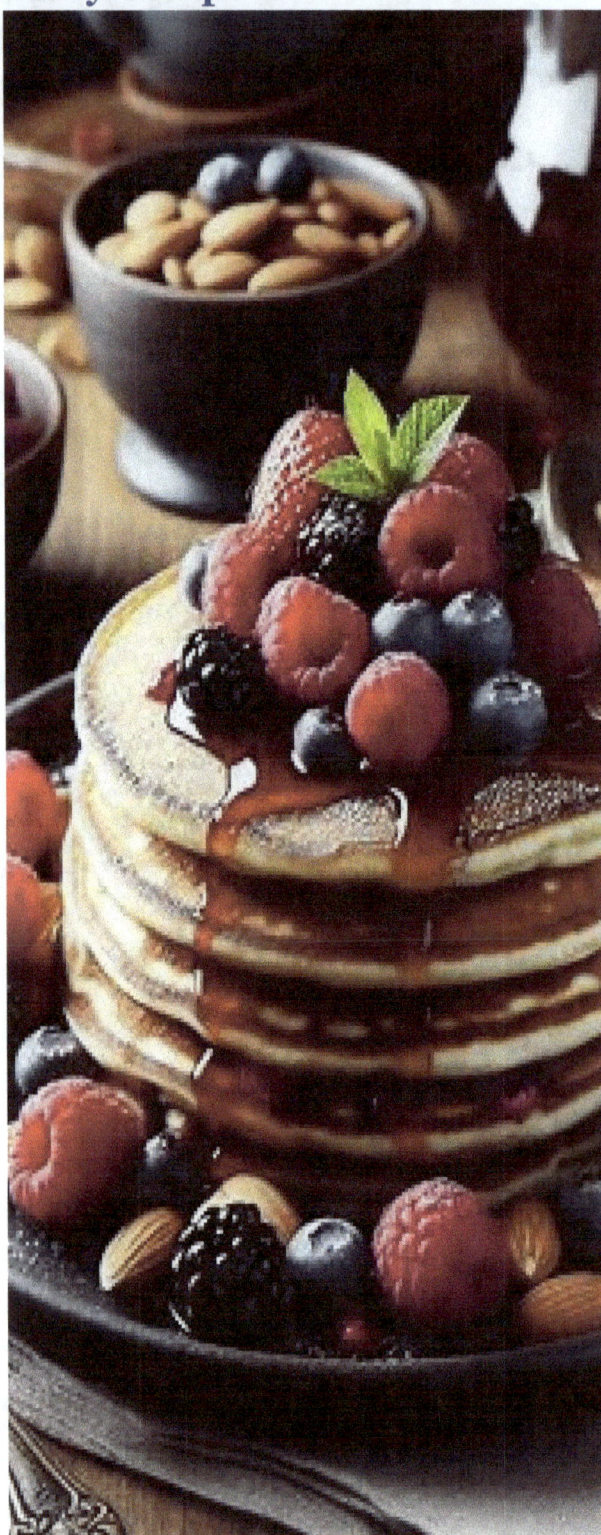

Prep Time: 5 minutes
Cooking Time: 10 minutes
Serves: 2
Ingredients:

- 1 cup almond flour
- 2 large eggs
- ½ cup unsweetened almond milk
- 1 teaspoon baking powder
- 1 teaspoon vanilla extract
- 1 teaspoon cinnamon
- 1 cup mixed berries (for compote)
- 1 teaspoon honey (for compote, optional)

Instructions:

1. In a bowl, whisk together almond flour, eggs, almond milk, baking powder, vanilla extract, and cinnamon until smooth.
2. Heat a non-stick skillet over medium heat and lightly grease with oil or butter.
3. Pour 1/4 cup of the pancake batter onto the skillet and cook for 2-3 minutes on each side, or until golden brown.
4. For the compote, heat the mixed berries in a small saucepan over medium heat for 5-7 minutes, adding honey if desired.
5. Serve the pancakes topped with the berry compote.

Nutritional Information (per serving):

- Calories: 300
- Protein: 12g
- Carbs: 15g
- Fiber: 5g
- Potassium: 200mg
- Sodium: 50mg

Tip: You can freeze leftover pancakes for a quick breakfast option during the week.

Rice Pudding with Vanilla and Stevia

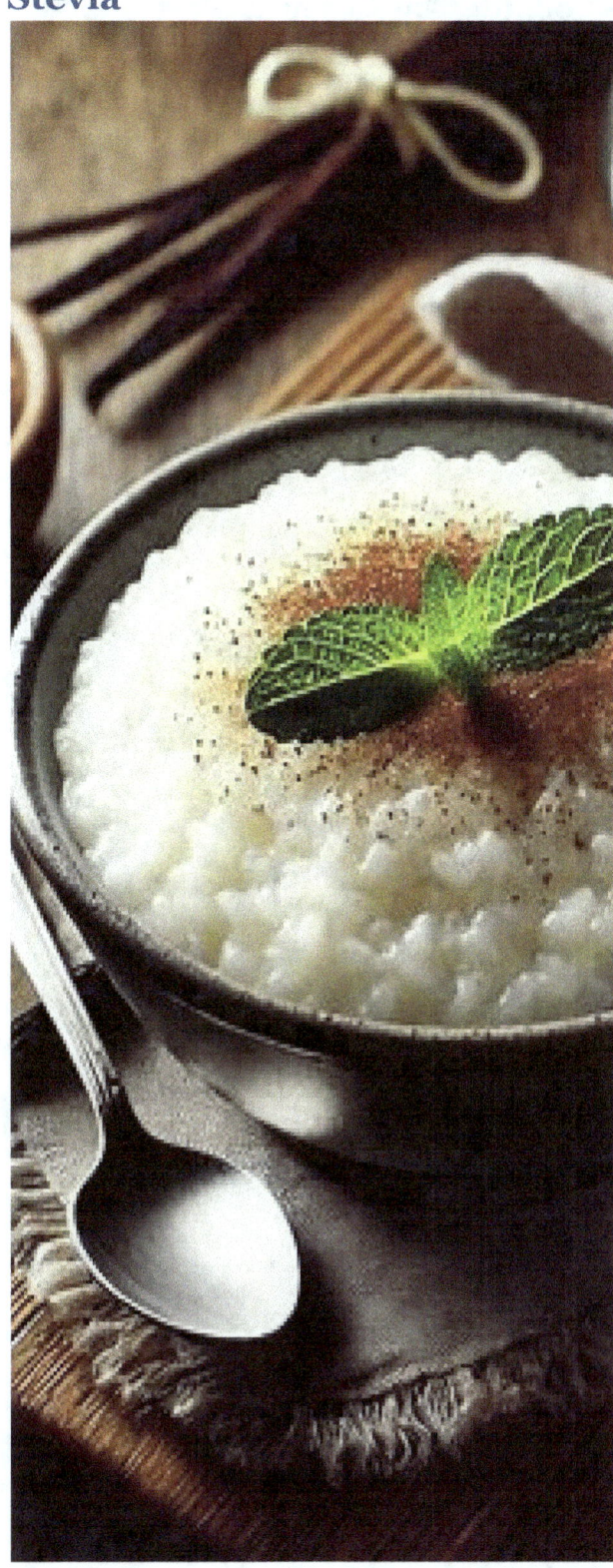

Prep Time: 5 minutes

Cooking Time: 20 minutes

Serves: 2

Ingredients:

- ½ cup white rice
- 1 ½ cups unsweetened almond milk
- 1 teaspoon vanilla extract
- 1-2 teaspoons stevia (or to taste)
- 1 teaspoon ground cinnamon (optional)

Instructions:

1. In a medium saucepan, bring the rice and almond milk to a boil.
2. Reduce the heat and simmer, stirring occasionally, for about 15-20 minutes until the rice is tender and the pudding thickens.
3. Stir in the vanilla extract, stevia, and cinnamon, if using.
4. Serve warm or chilled.

Nutritional Information (per serving):

- Calories: 180
- Protein: 3g
- Carbs: 35g
- Fiber: 1g
- Potassium: 150mg
- Sodium: 45mg

Tip: For a richer flavor, cook the rice with coconut milk instead of almond milk.

Rice Cakes with Almond Butter and Apple Slices

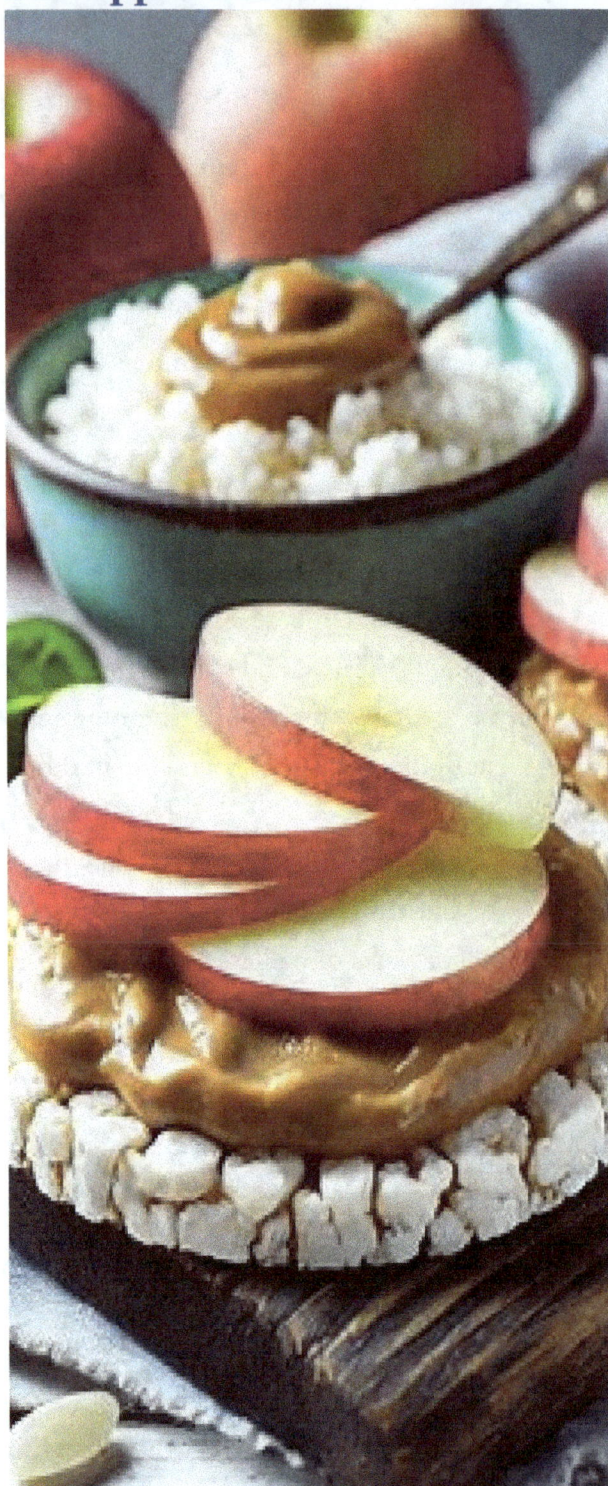

Prep Time: 5 minutes

Cooking Time: 0 minutes

Serves: 1

Ingredients:

- 2 plain rice cakes
- 2 tablespoons almond butter
- ½ apple, thinly sliced
- A sprinkle of cinnamon (optional)

Instructions:

1. Spread almond butter evenly over each rice cake.
2. Arrange apple slices on top of the almond butter.
3. Sprinkle with cinnamon, if desired, and serve.

Nutritional Information (per serving):

- Calories: 220
- Protein: 7g
- Carbs: 26g
- Fiber: 5g
- Potassium: 180mg
- Sodium: 30mg

Tip: You can substitute almond butter with peanut butter or sunflower seed butter for variety.

Cottage Cheese with Fresh Peaches and a Dash of Cinnamon

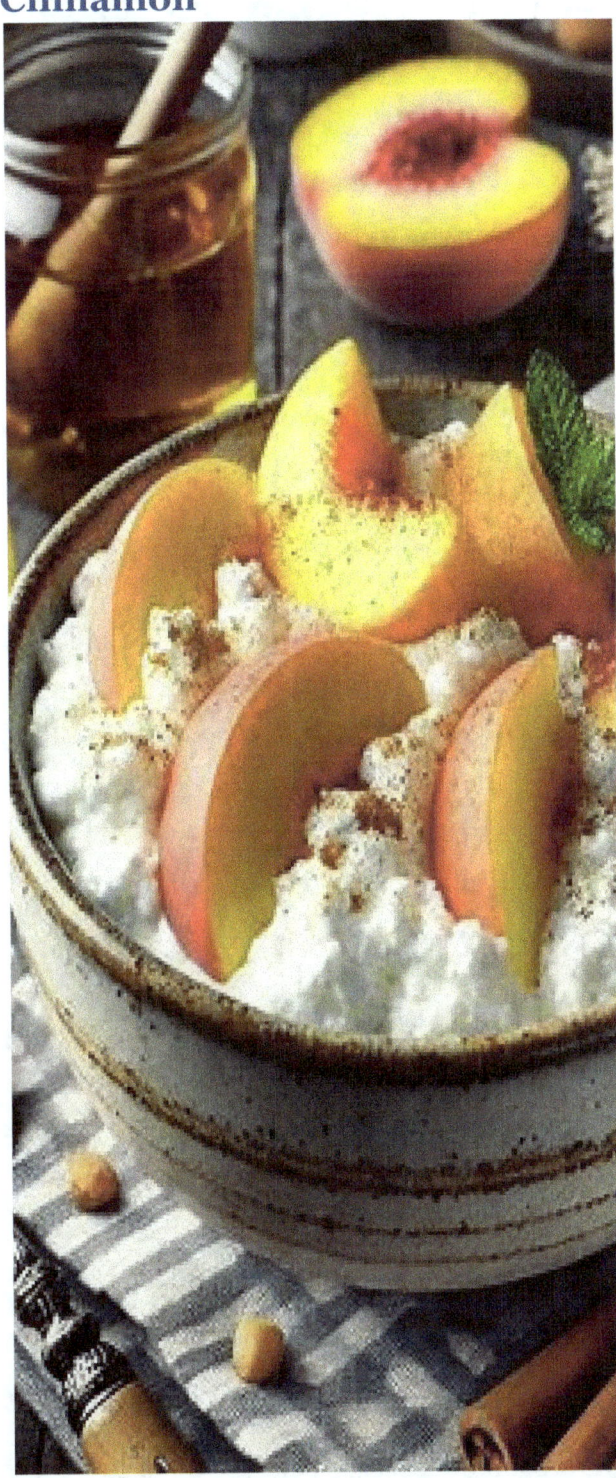

Prep Time: 5 minutes

Cooking Time: 0 minutes

Serves: 1

Ingredients:

- ½ cup low-fat cottage cheese
- 1 small peach, sliced
- ½ teaspoon cinnamon

Instructions:

1. Scoop the cottage cheese into a bowl.
2. Top with sliced peaches and a sprinkle of cinnamon.
3. Serve immediately.

Nutritional Information (per serving):

- Calories: 150
- Protein: 15g
- Carbs: 14g
- Fiber: 2g
- Potassium: 200mg
- Sodium: 400mg

Tip: Use fresh or frozen peaches for this recipe, depending on what is in season.

Low-Sodium Breakfast Burrito with Turkey and Spinach

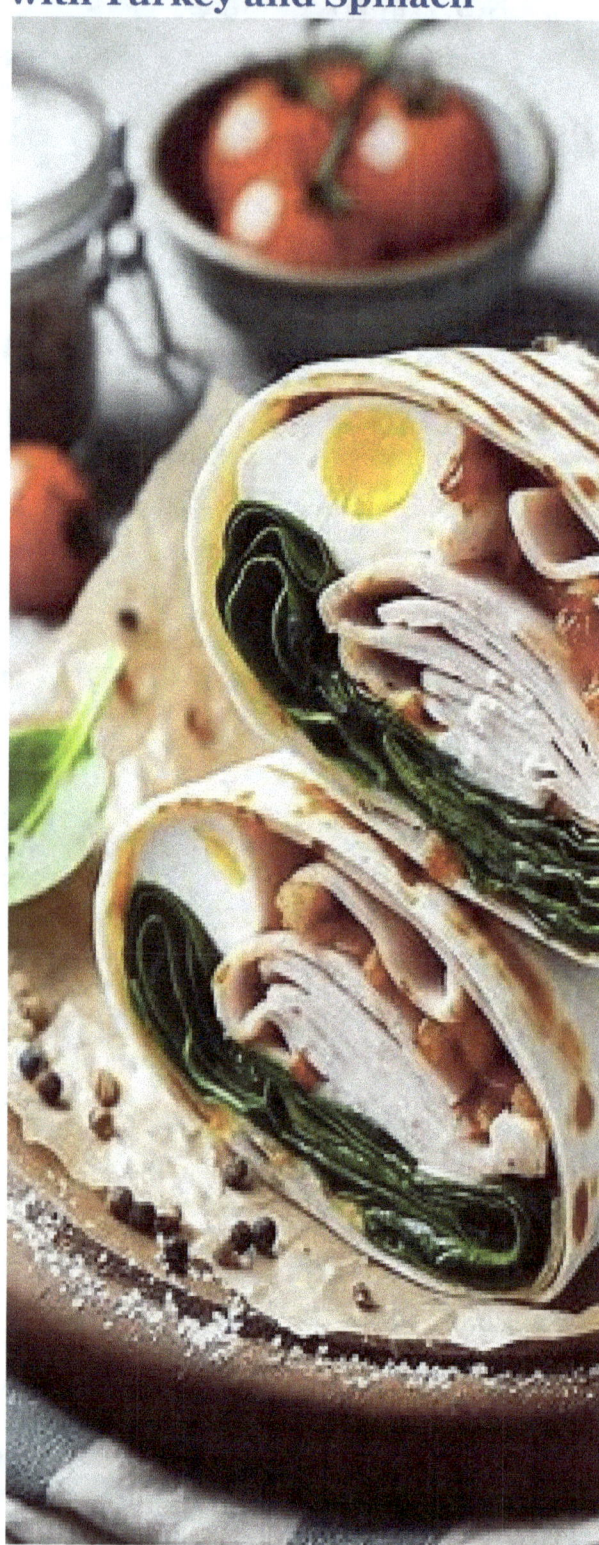

Prep Time: 10 minutes

Cooking Time: 10 minutes

Serves: 1

Ingredients:

- 1 whole wheat tortilla
- 2 oz cooked turkey breast, sliced
- 1/2 cup fresh spinach, chopped
- 1 large egg
- 1 tablespoon salsa (low-sodium)
- 1 teaspoon olive oil

Instructions:

1. Heat olive oil in a skillet over medium heat.
2. Scramble the egg in the skillet and cook until fully set.
3. Place the cooked turkey and spinach in the tortilla, followed by the scrambled egg and salsa.
4. Roll up the tortilla into a burrito and serve warm.

Nutritional Information (per serving):

- Calories: 280
- Protein: 25g
- Carbs: 25g
- Fiber: 4g
- Potassium: 400mg
- Sodium: 300mg

Tip: For added flavor, sprinkle with low-sodium cheese before rolling up the burrito.

Chapter 4
Lunches

Grilled Chicken Salad with Olive Oil and Lemon

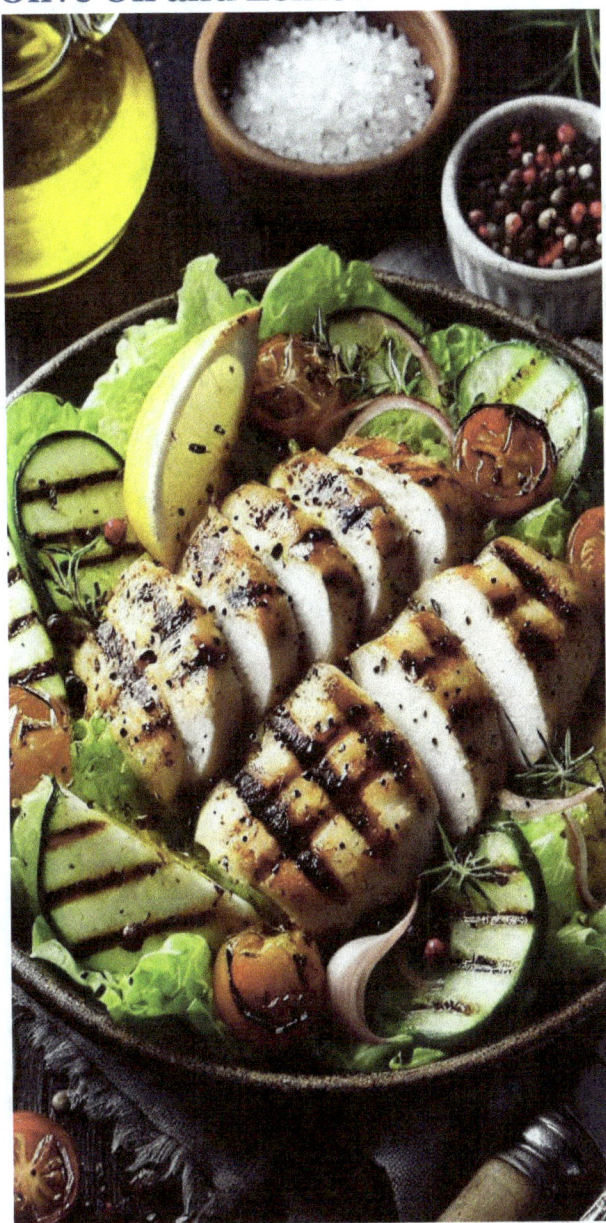

Serves: 2

Ingredients:

- 2 boneless, skinless chicken breasts
- 4 cups mixed greens (e.g., spinach, arugula, lettuce)
- 1 cucumber, thinly sliced
- 1 tablespoon olive oil
- 1 tablespoon lemon juice
- Salt and pepper to taste (use salt substitute if necessary)
- 1 teaspoon dried oregano
- 1 tablespoon fresh parsley, chopped (optional)

Instructions:

1. Preheat the grill or grill pan to medium-high heat.
2. Drizzle the chicken breasts with olive oil and season with oregano, salt, and pepper.
3. Grill the chicken for about 5-7 minutes per side, or until fully cooked (internal temperature should reach 165°F).
4. While the chicken is grilling, prepare the salad by combining the mixed greens and sliced cucumber in a large bowl.
5. Once the chicken is cooked, slice it into strips and add it to the salad.
6. Drizzle with lemon juice and toss gently.
7. Serve with a sprinkle of fresh parsley, if desired.

Nutritional Information (per serving):

- Calories: 280
- Protein: 35g
- Carbs: 10g
- Fiber: 4g
- Potassium: 450mg
- Sodium: 110mg

Tip: To make this salad even more filling, add a few slices of avocado (keeping potassium levels in mind).

Prep Time: 10 minutes
Cooking Time: 15 minutes

Quinoa and Cucumber Salad with Greek Yogurt Dressing

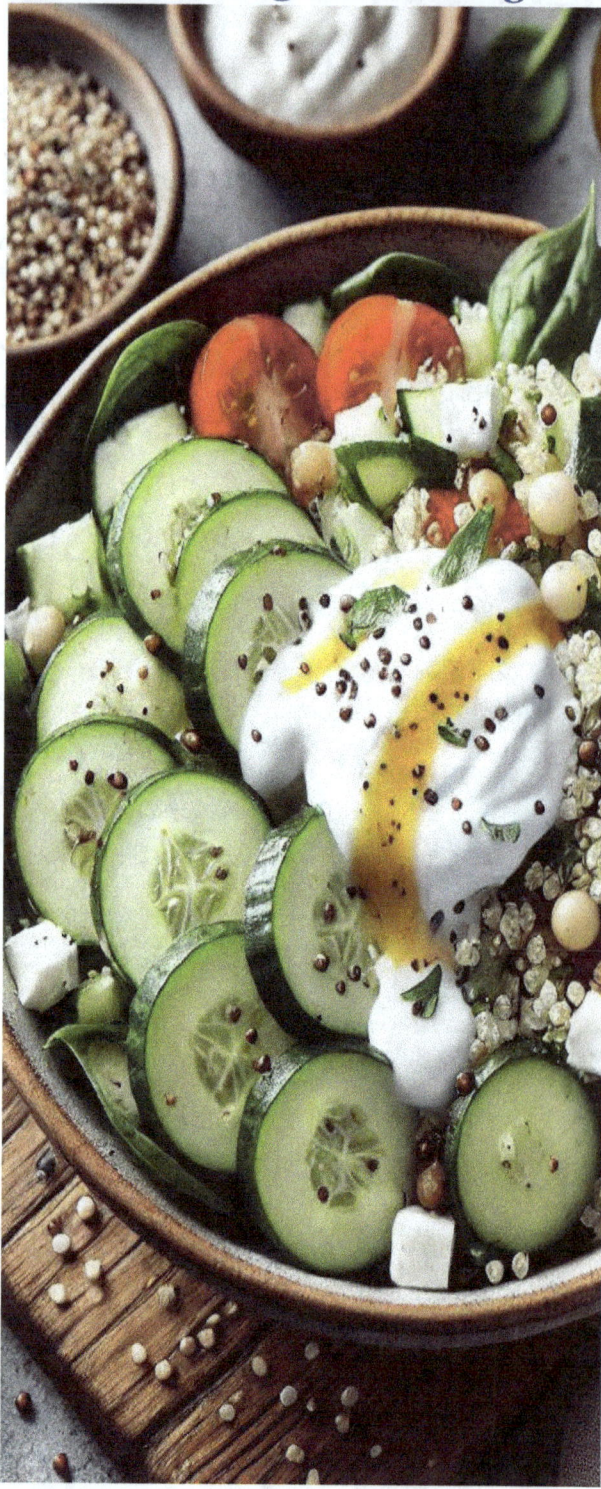

Serves: 2

Ingredients:

- 1 cup quinoa (uncooked)
- 1 cucumber, diced
- ¼ cup red onion, finely chopped
- ¼ cup fresh dill, chopped
- ½ cup plain Greek yogurt (low-fat)
- 1 tablespoon olive oil
- 1 tablespoon lemon juice
- Salt and pepper to taste (use salt substitute if necessary)

Instructions:

1. Rinse the quinoa under cold water.
2. In a saucepan, bring 2 cups of water to a boil. Add quinoa, reduce heat, and simmer for about 12-15 minutes, or until the quinoa is tender and the water is absorbed.
3. Let the quinoa cool for a few minutes, then fluff it with a fork.
4. In a bowl, combine the cooked quinoa, diced cucumber, red onion, and dill.
5. In a separate small bowl, whisk together the Greek yogurt, olive oil, lemon juice, and a pinch of salt and pepper.
6. Toss the quinoa salad with the yogurt dressing and serve chilled.

Nutritional Information (per serving):

- Calories: 250
- Protein: 9g
- Carbs: 35g
- Fiber: 4g
- Potassium: 300mg
- Sodium: 120mg

Tip: For added crunch, top with some toasted sunflower seeds or pumpkin seeds.

Prep Time: 15 minutes
Cooking Time: 15 minutes

Vegetable Soup (Low-Sodium)

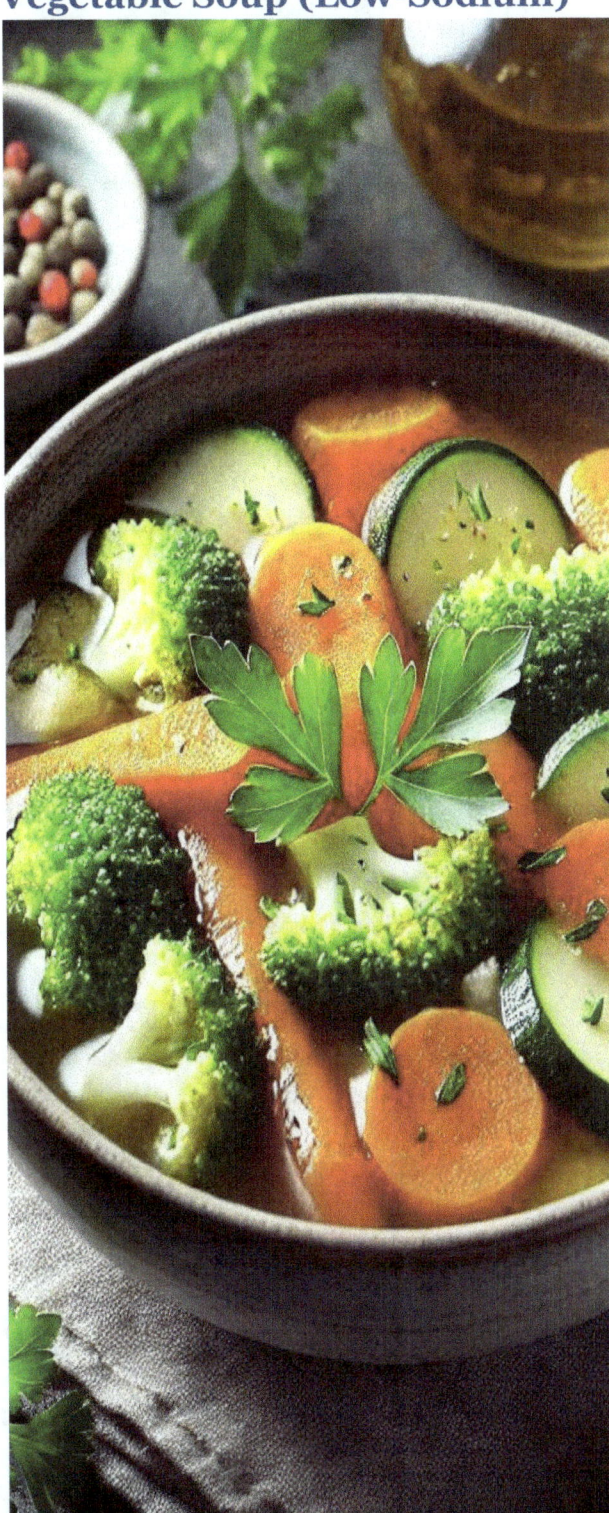

Prep Time: 10 minutes
Cooking Time: 30 minutes
Serves: 4
Ingredients:

- 2 tablespoons olive oil
- 1 small onion, diced
- 2 carrots, peeled and chopped
- 1 celery stalk, chopped
- 2 cups low-sodium vegetable broth
- 1 zucchini, chopped
- 1 cup green beans, chopped
- 1 teaspoon dried thyme
- Salt and pepper to taste (use salt substitute if necessary)

Instructions:

1. Heat olive oil in a large pot over medium heat.
2. Add the onion, carrots, and celery and sauté for about 5 minutes until softened.
3. Add the vegetable broth, zucchini, green beans, and thyme.
4. Bring to a boil, then reduce heat and simmer for 20 minutes or until the vegetables are tender.
5. Season with salt and pepper, and serve hot.

Nutritional Information (per serving):

- Calories: 120
- Protein: 3g
- Carbs: 20g
- Fiber: 5g
- Potassium: 450mg
- Sodium: 50mg

Tip: This soup can be made in bulk and stored in the fridge for up to 3 days or frozen for longer storage.

Lentil Salad with Cherry Tomatoes and Parsley

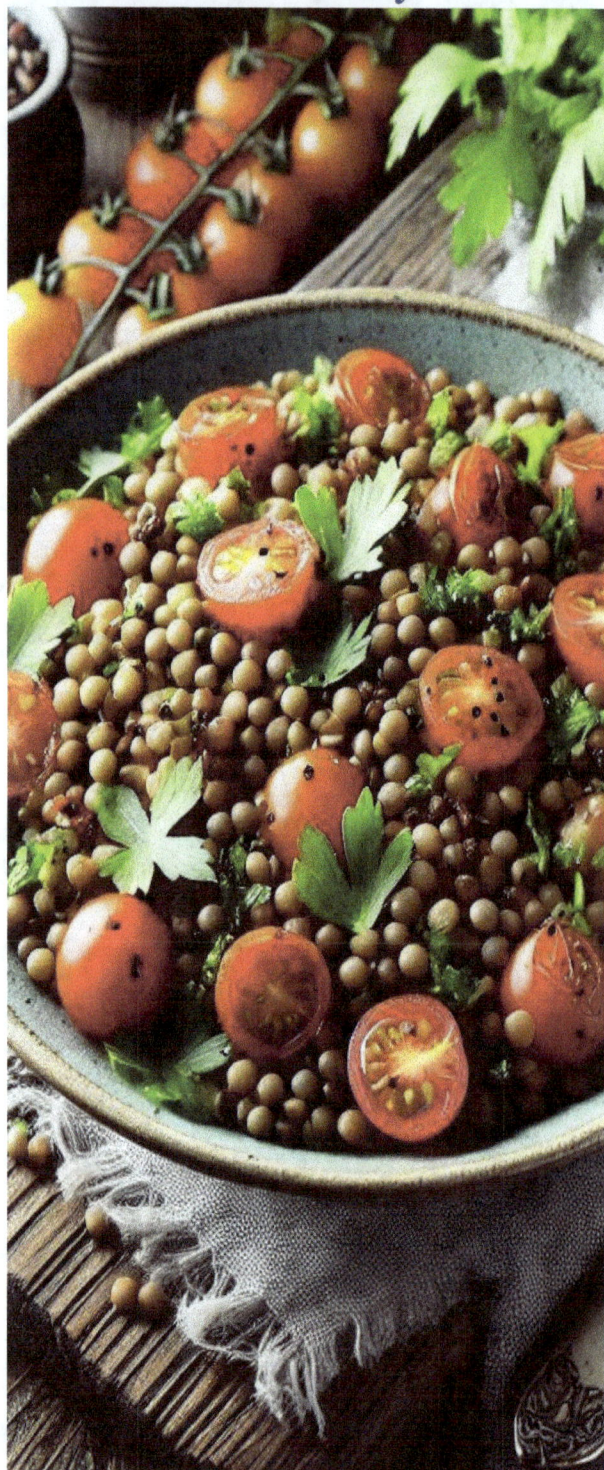

Prep Time: 10 minutes
Cooking Time: 25 minutes
Serves: 2
Ingredients:

- 1 cup dried lentils, rinsed
- 1 pint cherry tomatoes, halved
- ¼ cup fresh parsley, chopped
- 2 tablespoons olive oil
- 1 tablespoon lemon juice
- Salt and pepper to taste (use salt substitute if necessary)

Instructions:

1. In a pot, bring 3 cups of water to a boil and add the lentils.
2. Reduce heat and simmer for about 25 minutes or until the lentils are tender. Drain any excess water.
3. Let the lentils cool slightly, then transfer them to a bowl.
4. Add the cherry tomatoes and chopped parsley.
5. Drizzle with olive oil and lemon juice, then toss everything together.
6. Season with salt and pepper and serve.

Nutritional Information (per serving):

- Calories: 250
- Protein: 15g
- Carbs: 40g
- Fiber: 12g
- Potassium: 350mg
- Sodium: 80mg

Tip: For a more filling salad, add a handful of arugula or spinach.

Rice and Bean Bowl with Roasted Veggies

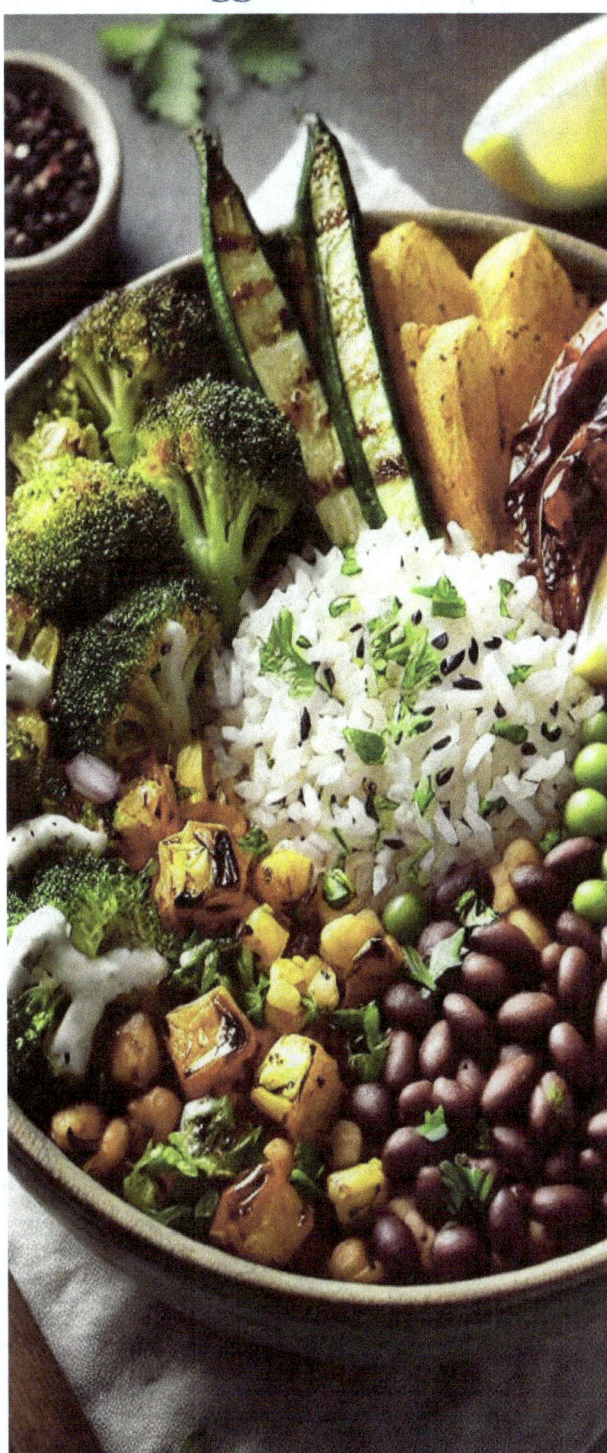

Prep Time: 10 minutes
Cooking Time: 30 minutes
Serves: 2
Ingredients:

- 1 cup cooked brown rice
- 1 cup cooked black beans (or kidney beans)
- 1 zucchini, chopped
- 1 red bell pepper, chopped
- 1 tablespoon olive oil
- 1 teaspoon cumin
- 1 teaspoon smoked paprika
- Salt and pepper to taste (use salt substitute if necessary)

Instructions:

1. Preheat the oven to 400°F (200°C).
2. Toss the zucchini and bell pepper in olive oil, cumin, smoked paprika, salt, and pepper.
3. Spread the vegetables in a single layer on a baking sheet and roast for 20-25 minutes, or until tender.
4. In a bowl, combine the cooked rice and beans.
5. Top with the roasted veggies and serve.

Nutritional Information (per serving):

- Calories: 350
- Protein: 12g
- Carbs: 60g
- Fiber: 10g
- Potassium: 650mg
- Sodium: 70mg

Tip: For a little extra flavor, drizzle with some fresh lime juice before serving.

Tuna Salad with Cabbage and Light Mayo

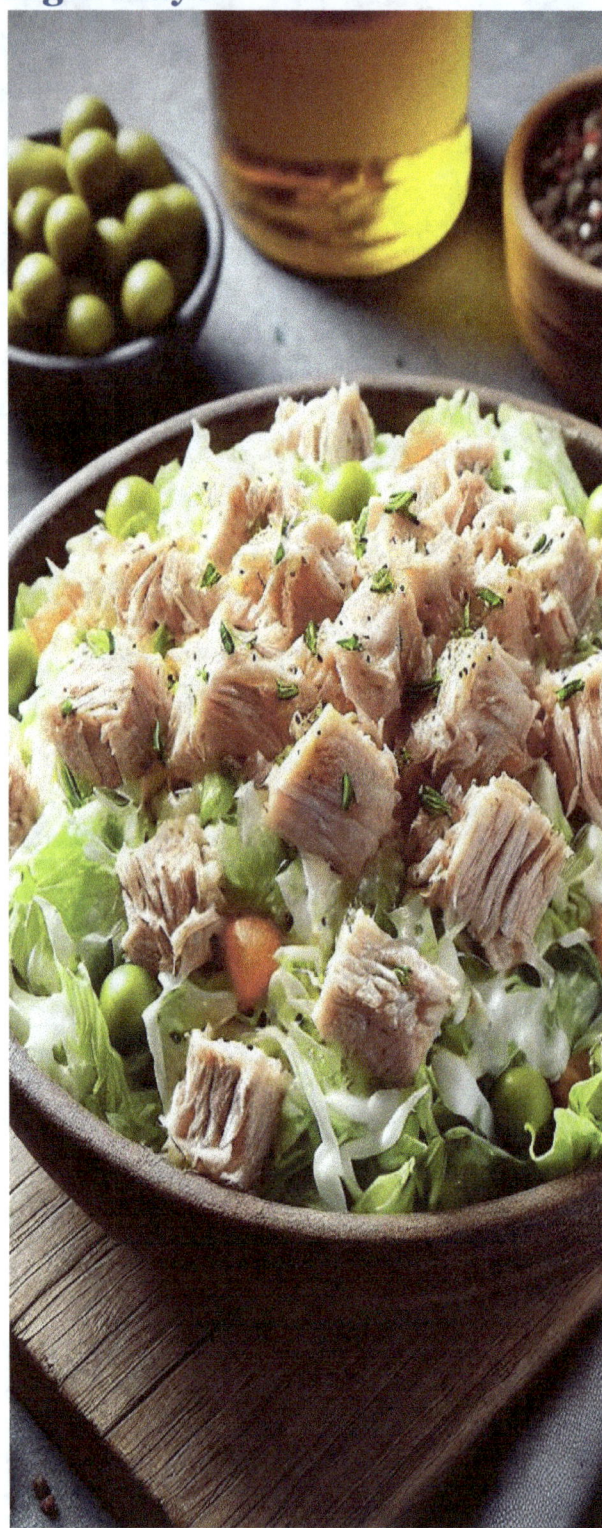

Prep Time: 10 minutes

Cooking Time: 0 minutes

Serves: 2

Ingredients:

- 1 can tuna (in water), drained
- 2 cups cabbage, shredded
- 2 tablespoons light mayonnaise
- 1 tablespoon Dijon mustard
- Salt and pepper to taste (use salt substitute if necessary)

Instructions:

1. In a large bowl, combine the tuna and shredded cabbage.
2. In a small bowl, whisk together the light mayonnaise, Dijon mustard, and salt and pepper.
3. Add the dressing to the tuna and cabbage mixture and toss to coat.
4. Serve chilled.

Nutritional Information (per serving):

- Calories: 250
- Protein: 30g
- Carbs: 10g
- Fiber: 4g
- Potassium: 300mg
- Sodium: 200mg

Tip: Add some sliced cucumber or bell peppers for extra crunch.

Stuffed Bell Peppers with Ground Turkey and Quinoa

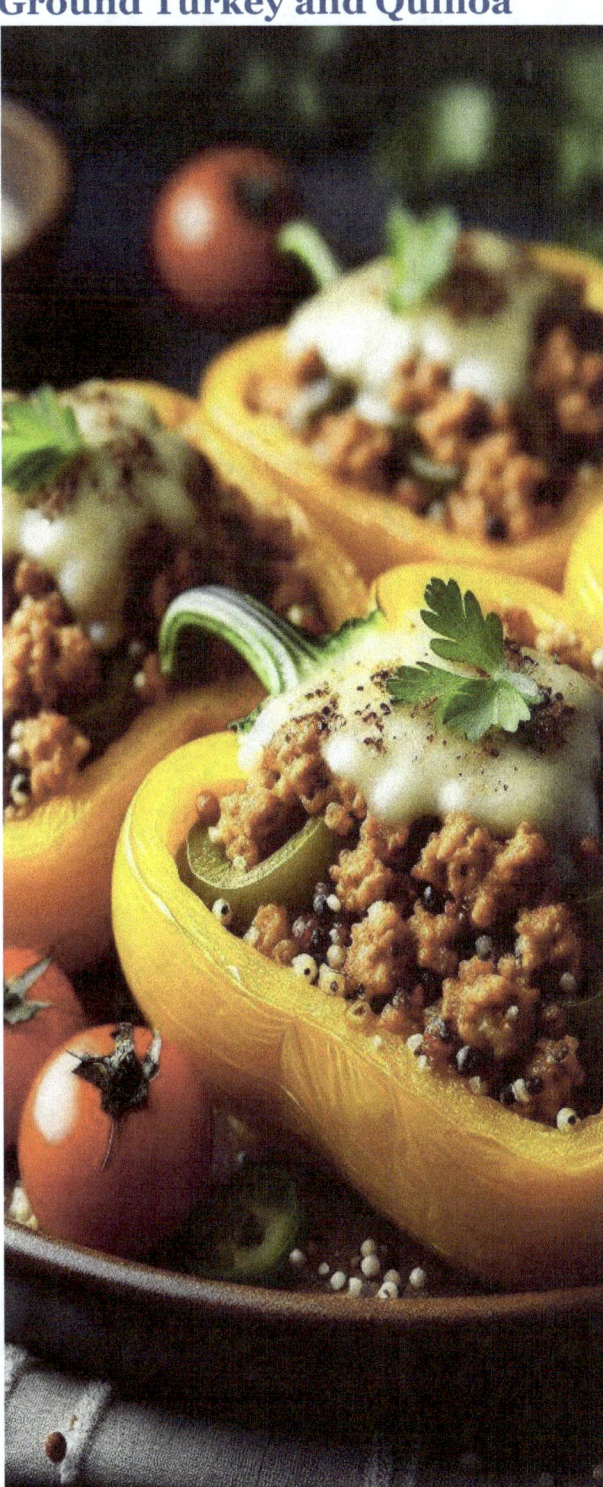

Prep Time: 15 minutes
Cooking Time: 35 minutes
Serves: 2
Ingredients:

- 2 bell peppers, halved and seeded
- 1/2 pound ground turkey
- 1/2 cup cooked quinoa
- 1 small onion, diced
- 1 tablespoon olive oil
- 1 teaspoon garlic powder
- Salt and pepper to taste (use salt substitute if necessary)

Instructions:

1. Preheat the oven to 375°F (190°C).
2. In a skillet, heat olive oil over medium heat. Add the ground turkey and cook until browned.
3. Stir in the cooked quinoa, onion, garlic powder, salt, and pepper.
4. Stuff the bell pepper halves with the turkey-quinoa mixture and place them in a baking dish.
5. Cover with foil and bake for 30 minutes.

Nutritional Information (per serving):

- Calories: 320
- Protein: 35g
- Carbs: 25g
- Fiber: 6g
- Potassium: 600mg
- Sodium: 180mg

Tip: Add a sprinkle of low-sodium cheese on top before baking for extra flavor.

Chickpea and Spinach Stir Fry

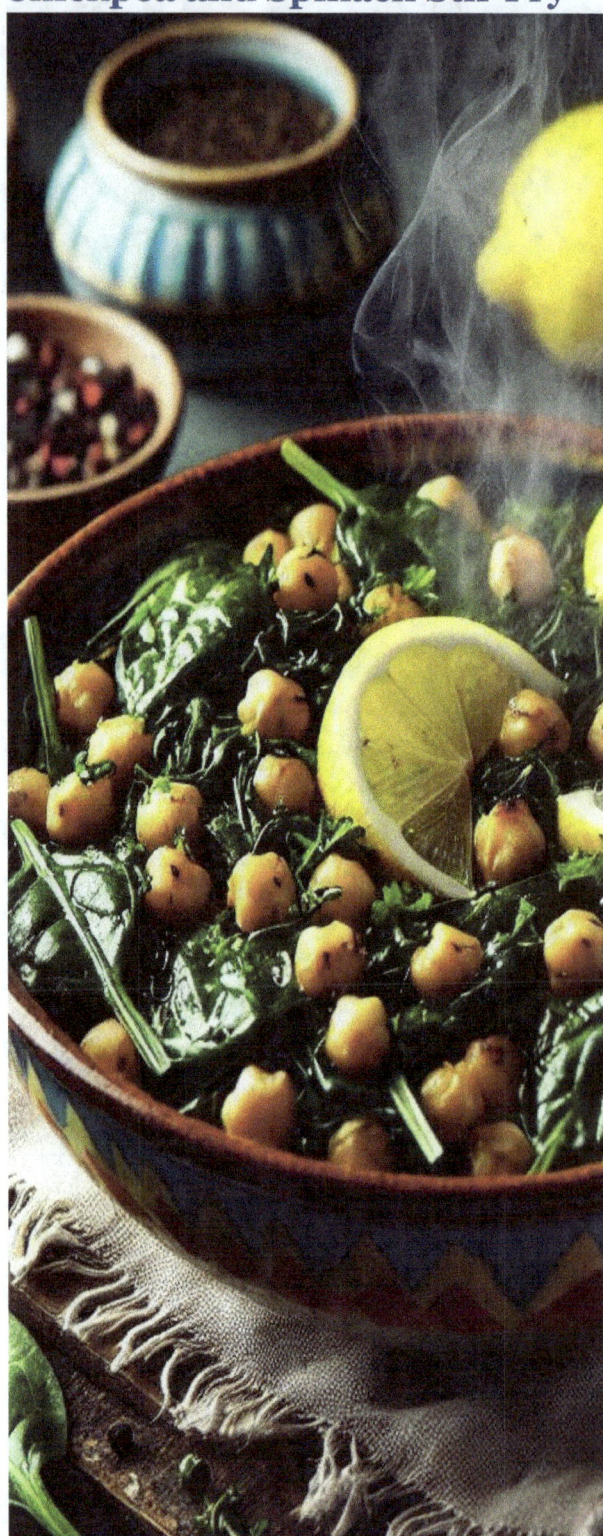

Prep Time: 10 minutes
Cooking Time: 15 minutes
Serves: 2
Ingredients:

- 1 can chickpeas (low-sodium, drained and rinsed)
- 2 cups fresh spinach, chopped
- 1 tablespoon olive oil
- 1 tablespoon garlic, minced
- 1 teaspoon cumin
- 1 teaspoon turmeric
- 1 tablespoon lemon juice
- Salt and pepper to taste (use salt substitute if necessary)

Instructions:

1. Heat olive oil in a large skillet or wok over medium heat.
2. Add the garlic and sauté for 1-2 minutes until fragrant.
3. Add the chickpeas to the skillet, stirring occasionally, for about 5 minutes, allowing them to crisp up slightly.
4. Stir in the cumin, turmeric, salt, and pepper.
5. Add the chopped spinach and cook for 2-3 minutes until wilted.
6. Drizzle with lemon juice and serve warm.

Nutritional Information (per serving):

- Calories: 250
- Protein: 12g
- Carbs: 38g
- Fiber: 10g
- Potassium: 450mg
- Sodium: 120mg

Tip: Serve this stir-fry with a side of brown rice or quinoa for a more filling meal.

Egg Salad on Whole Grain Toast

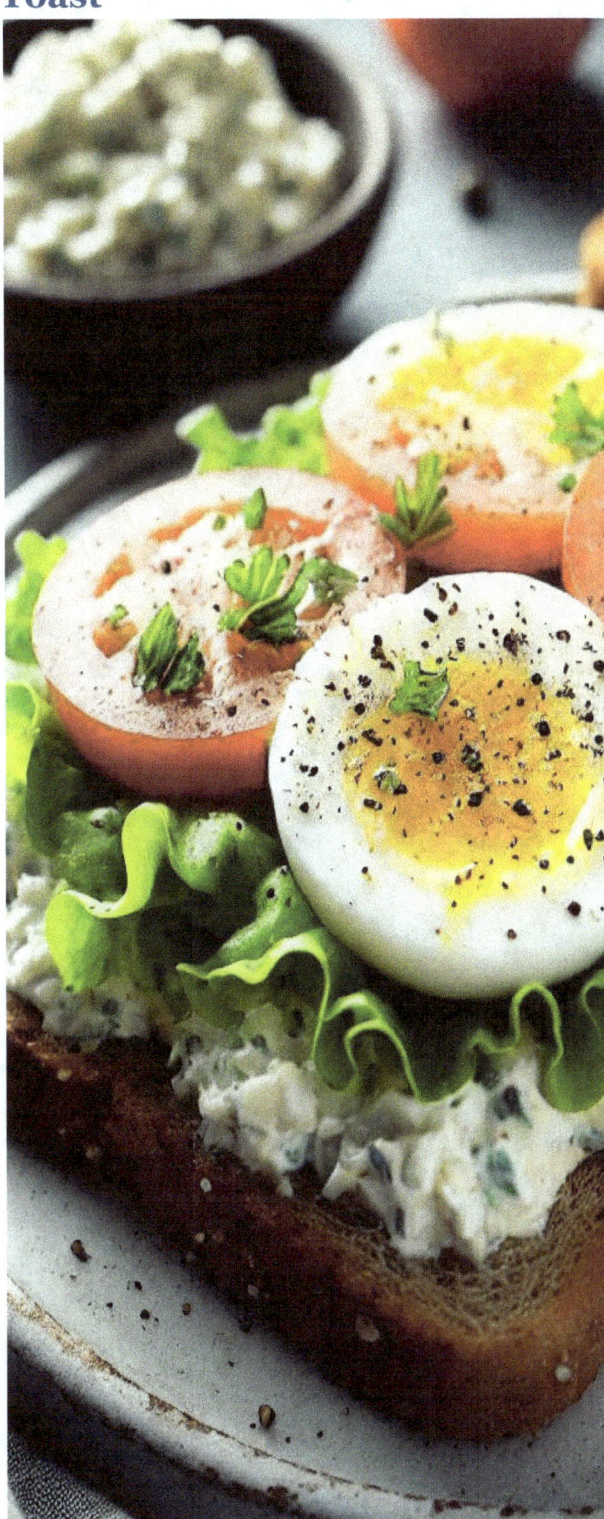

Prep Time: 10 minutes
Cooking Time: 10 minutes
Serves: 2
Ingredients:

- 4 large eggs, hard-boiled
- 2 tablespoons light mayonnaise
- 1 tablespoon Dijon mustard
- 1 teaspoon fresh dill, chopped
- 2 slices whole grain bread (toasted)
- Salt and pepper to taste (use salt substitute if necessary)

Instructions:

1. Peel and chop the hard-boiled eggs into small pieces.
2. In a small bowl, mix the eggs with mayonnaise, Dijon mustard, dill, salt, and pepper.
3. Toast the whole grain bread and spread the egg salad evenly on each slice.
4. Serve immediately.

Nutritional Information (per serving):

- Calories: 300
- Protein: 18g
- Carbs: 22g
- Fiber: 4g
- Potassium: 300mg
- Sodium: 200mg

Tip: For added crunch, top with some fresh cucumber or lettuce.

Grilled Salmon with Steamed Broccoli and Brown Rice

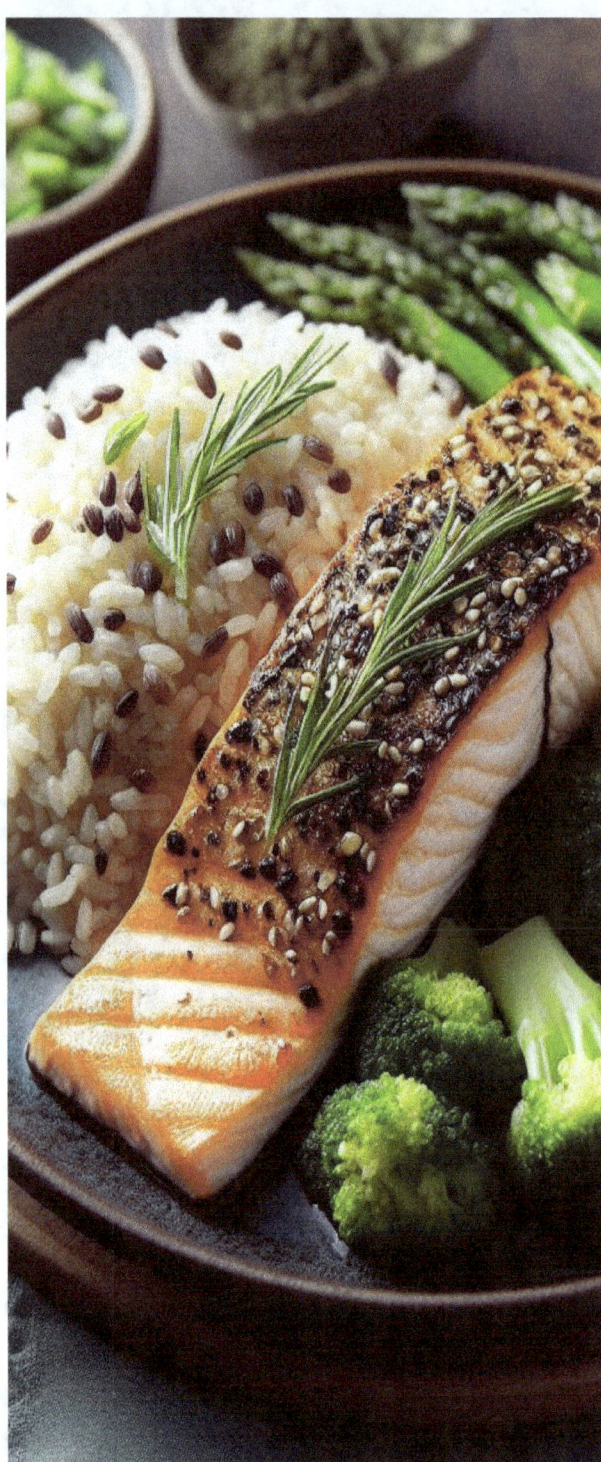

Prep Time: 10 minutes
Cooking Time: 20 minutes
Serves: 2
Ingredients:

- 2 salmon fillets (4-6 oz each)
- 1 cup broccoli florets
- 1 cup cooked brown rice
- 1 tablespoon olive oil
- 1 teaspoon lemon juice
- Salt and pepper to taste (use salt substitute if necessary)
- 1 tablespoon fresh parsley, chopped

Instructions:

1. Preheat the grill or grill pan to medium-high heat.
2. Drizzle the salmon fillets with olive oil, lemon juice, salt, and pepper.
3. Grill the salmon for 4-5 minutes on each side, or until it flakes easily with a fork.
4. Meanwhile, steam the broccoli for 5-7 minutes until tender.
5. Serve the grilled salmon with steamed broccoli and a side of brown rice.
6. Garnish with fresh parsley.

Nutritional Information (per serving):

- Calories: 400
- Protein: 35g
- Carbs: 40g
- Fiber: 6g
- Potassium: 800mg
- Sodium: 150mg

Tip: To make the meal even more flavorful, drizzle the salmon with a little bit of balsamic glaze.

Cauliflower Rice with Tofu and Peas

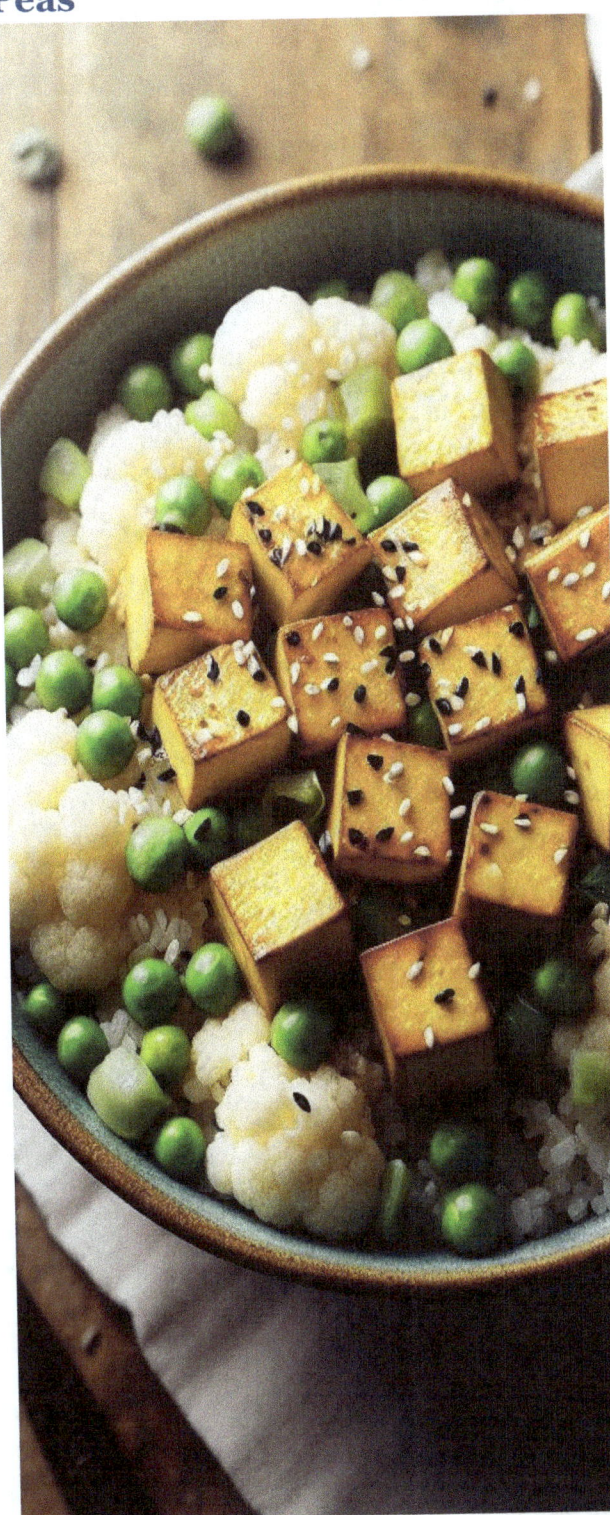

Prep Time: 10 minutes
Cooking Time: 15 minutes
Serves: 2
Ingredients:

- 1 small cauliflower head, grated into rice-sized pieces (or use pre-made cauliflower rice)
- 1 block firm tofu, drained and cubed
- 1 cup frozen peas
- 1 tablespoon olive oil
- 1 tablespoon soy sauce (low-sodium)
- 1 teaspoon sesame oil (optional)
- Salt and pepper to taste (use salt substitute if necessary)

Instructions:

1. Heat olive oil in a large skillet over medium heat.
2. Add the cubed tofu and cook for 5-7 minutes until golden brown.
3. Add the cauliflower rice to the skillet and cook for 3-4 minutes until it starts to soften.
4. Stir in the frozen peas, soy sauce, sesame oil (if using), salt, and pepper.
5. Cook for an additional 3-4 minutes, then serve warm.

Nutritional Information (per serving):

- Calories: 250
- Protein: 18g
- Carbs: 18g
- Fiber: 6g
- Potassium: 600mg
- Sodium: 250mg

Tip: For added crunch, top with some chopped almonds or sunflower seeds.

Zucchini Noodles with Avocado and Pesto

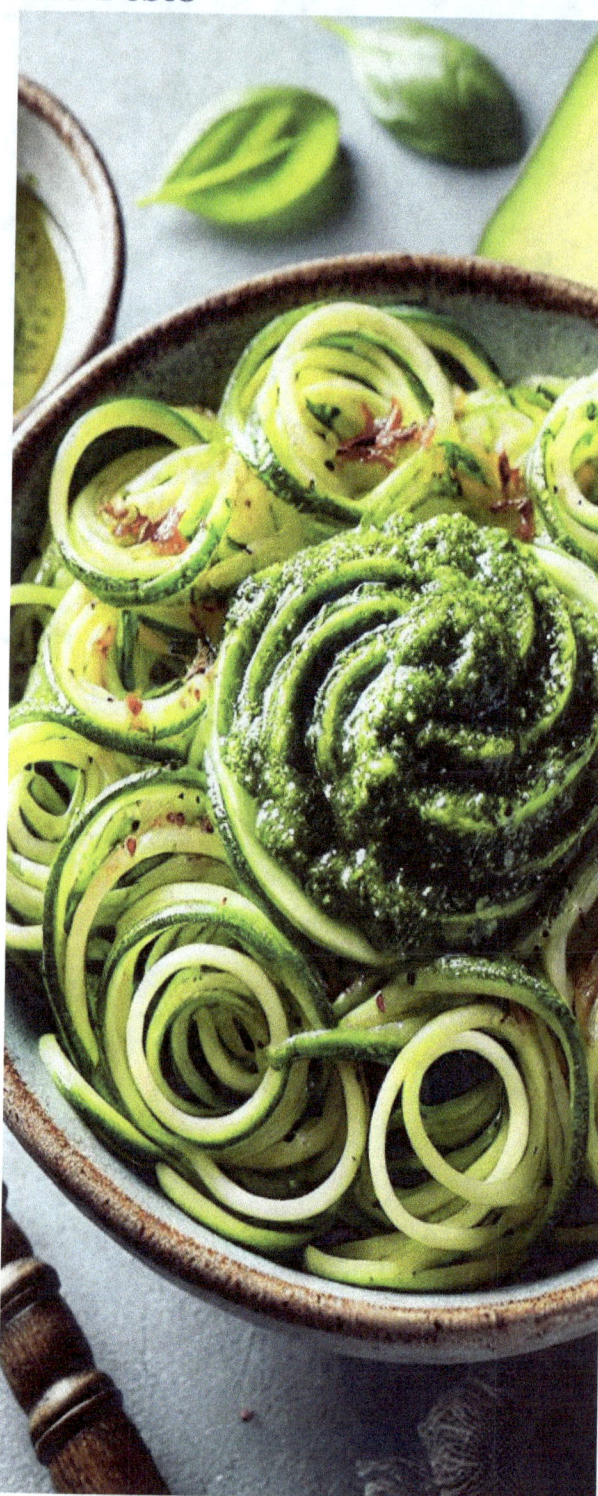

Prep Time: 15 minutes
Cooking Time: 5 minutes
Serves: 2
Ingredients:

- 2 medium zucchinis, spiralized into noodles
- 1 ripe avocado, pitted and peeled
- 1/4 cup fresh basil leaves
- 1 tablespoon lemon juice
- 2 tablespoons olive oil
- 1 tablespoon nutritional yeast (optional)
- Salt and pepper to taste (use salt substitute if necessary)

Instructions:

1. Spiralize the zucchinis into noodles using a spiralizer or julienne peeler.
2. In a blender or food processor, combine the avocado, basil, lemon juice, olive oil, nutritional yeast, salt, and pepper.
3. Blend until smooth to make the pesto.
4. Toss the zucchini noodles with the avocado pesto until fully coated.
5. Serve immediately.

Nutritional Information (per serving):

- Calories: 300
- Protein: 4g
- Carbs: 20g
- Fiber: 7g
- Potassium: 700mg
- Sodium: 150mg

Tip: If you prefer a more "noodle-like" texture, lightly sauté the zucchini noodles in olive oil for 2-3 minutes before tossing them with the pesto.

Chicken and Sweet Potato Stew

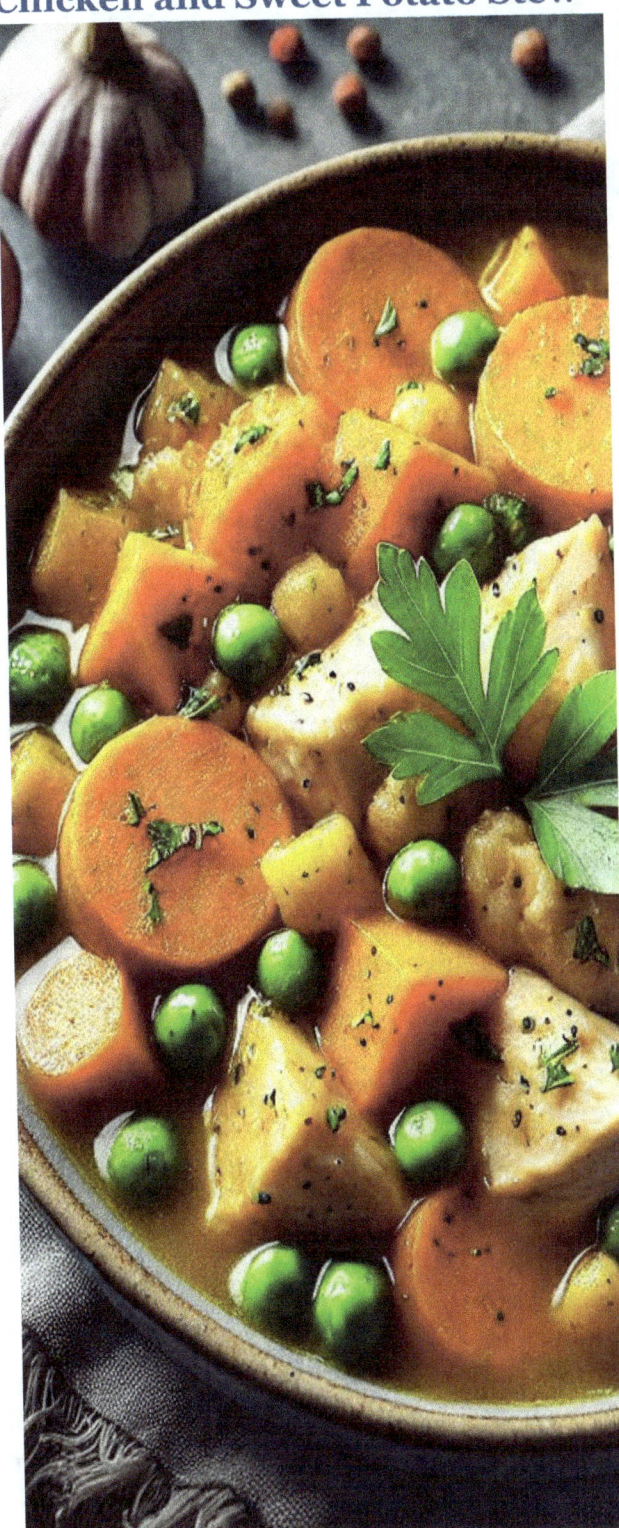

Prep Time: 10 minutes
Cooking Time: 30 minutes
Serves: 4
Ingredients:

- 2 boneless, skinless chicken breasts, cubed
- 2 medium sweet potatoes, peeled and chopped
- 2 cups low-sodium chicken broth
- 1 teaspoon ground turmeric
- 1 teaspoon cinnamon
- 1 tablespoon olive oil
- 2 cups spinach, chopped
- Salt and pepper to taste (use salt substitute if necessary)

Instructions:

1. In a large pot, heat olive oil over medium heat.
2. Add the cubed chicken and cook until browned, about 5-7 minutes.
3. Add the sweet potatoes, chicken broth, turmeric, cinnamon, salt, and pepper.
4. Bring to a boil, then reduce heat and simmer for 20 minutes or until the sweet potatoes are tender.
5. Stir in the spinach and cook for an additional 2-3 minutes until wilted.
6. Serve warm.

Nutritional Information (per serving):

- Calories: 320
- Protein: 28g
- Carbs: 30g
- Fiber: 6g
- Potassium: 800mg
- Sodium: 150mg

Tip: This stew freezes well, so consider making extra for easy meal prep.

Low-Sodium Hummus and Veggie Wrap

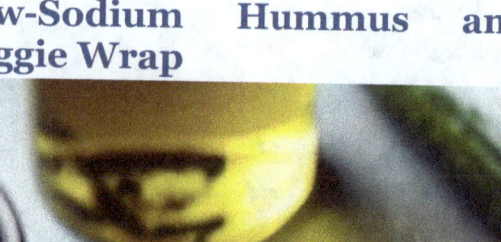

Prep Time: 10 minutes
Cooking Time: 0 minutes
Serves: 2
Ingredients:

- 2 whole grain tortillas
- 1/4 cup low-sodium hummus
- 1 cucumber, sliced
- 1 carrot, grated
- 1/2 bell pepper, thinly sliced
- 2 tablespoons fresh cilantro, chopped
- Salt and pepper to taste (use salt substitute if necessary)

Instructions:

1. Spread hummus evenly on each tortilla.
2. Arrange the cucumber, carrot, bell pepper, and cilantro on top of the hummus.
3. Sprinkle with salt and pepper.
4. Roll up the tortilla and serve.

Nutritional Information (per serving):

- Calories: 250
- Protein: 6g
- Carbs: 40g
- Fiber: 8g
- Potassium: 400mg
- Sodium: 150mg

Tip: For extra crunch, try adding some chopped radishes or alfalfa sprouts.

Toasted Veggie Sandwich with Sunflower Seed Butter

Prep Time: 10 minutes
Cooking Time: 5 minutes
Serves: 2
Ingredients:

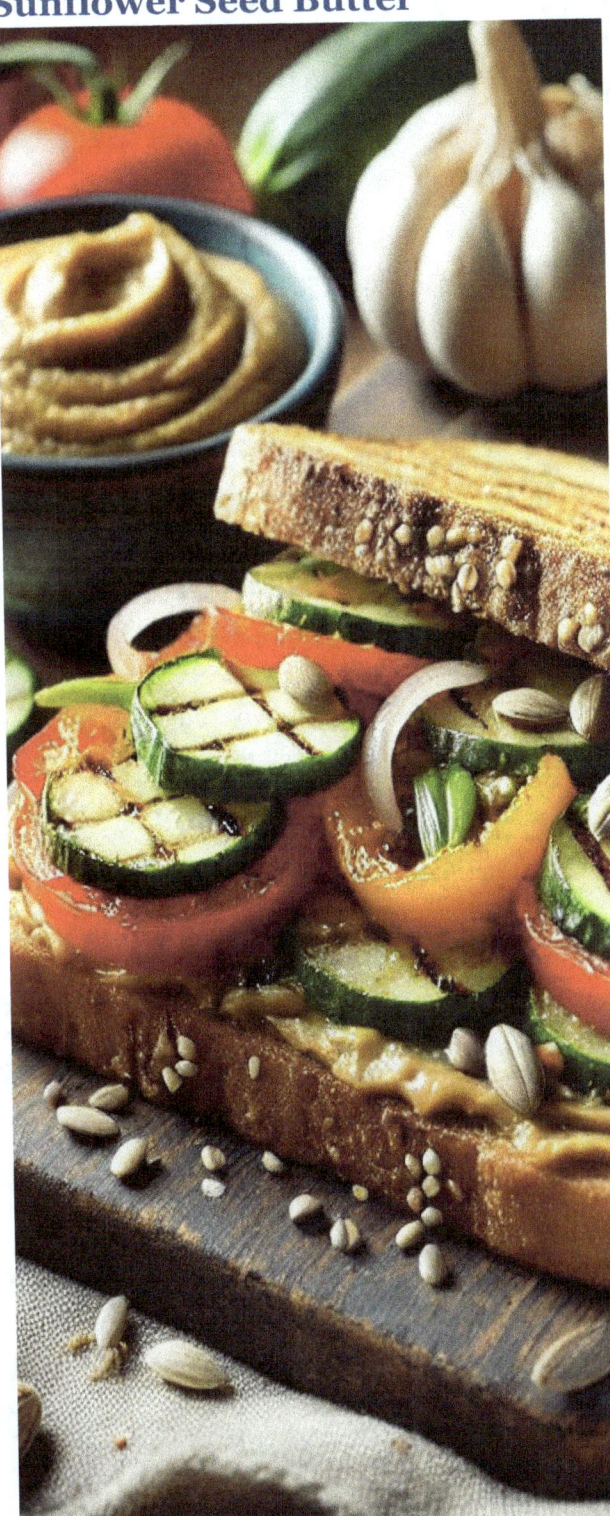

- 2 slices whole grain bread
- 2 tablespoons sunflower seed butter
- 1/2 cucumber, sliced
- 1/2 avocado, sliced
- 1/4 cup shredded carrots
- 1 tablespoon lemon juice
- Salt and pepper to taste (use salt substitute if necessary)

Instructions:

1. Toast the slices of whole grain bread.
2. Spread sunflower seed butter on each slice of toast.
3. Layer the cucumber, avocado, and shredded carrots on top of one slice of bread.
4. Drizzle with lemon juice and season with salt and pepper.
5. Top with the second slice of bread to form a sandwich.
6. Serve immediately.

Nutritional Information (per serving):

- Calories: 300
- Protein: 9g
- Carbs: 34g
- Fiber: 8g
- Potassium: 500mg
- Sodium: 120mg

Tip: For an extra burst of flavor, you can add some fresh basil or spinach leaves to the sandwich.

Chapter 5
Dinners

Baked Lemon Herb Salmon with Roasted Asparagus

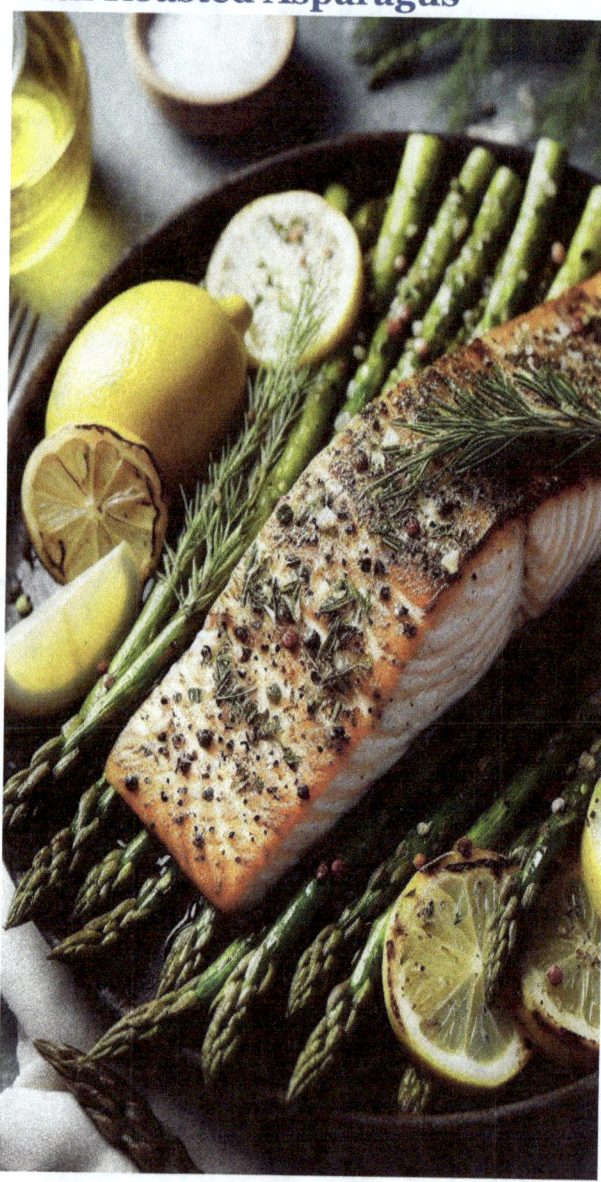

Serves: 2

Ingredients:

- 2 salmon fillets (4-6 oz each)
- 1 bunch asparagus, trimmed
- 1 tablespoon olive oil
- 1 tablespoon lemon juice
- 1 teaspoon dried rosemary
- 1 teaspoon garlic powder
- Salt and pepper to taste (use salt substitute if necessary)

Instructions:

1. Preheat your oven to 400°F (200°C).
2. Place the salmon fillets on a baking sheet lined with parchment paper.
3. Drizzle the salmon with olive oil and lemon juice. Sprinkle rosemary, garlic powder, salt, and pepper over the fillets.
4. Arrange the asparagus around the salmon and drizzle with a bit of olive oil, salt, and pepper.
5. Bake for 20-25 minutes, or until the salmon is cooked through and the asparagus is tender.
6. Serve immediately.

Nutritional Information (per serving):

- Calories: 350
- Protein: 35g
- Carbs: 10g
- Fiber: 4g
- Potassium: 850mg
- Sodium: 150mg

Prep Time: 10 minutes
Cooking Time: 25 minutes

Tip: You can also grill the salmon for a smoky flavor and quicker cooking time.

Chicken Stir-Fry with Bell Peppers and Zucchini

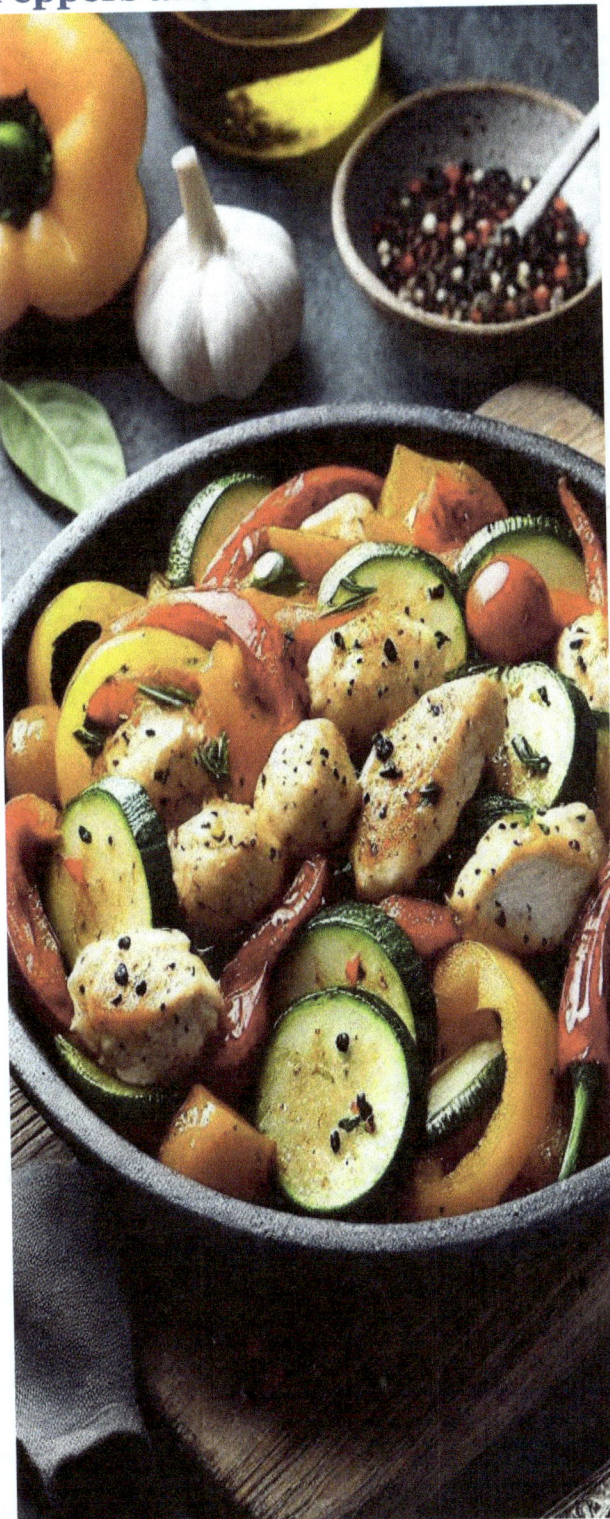

Prep Time: 15 minutes
Cooking Time: 10 minutes
Serves: 2
Ingredients:

- 2 chicken breasts, thinly sliced
- 1 bell pepper, sliced
- 1 zucchini, sliced
- 1 tablespoon olive oil
- 2 tablespoons low-sodium soy sauce
- 1 tablespoon rice vinegar
- 1 teaspoon sesame oil
- 1 teaspoon garlic, minced
- 1 teaspoon fresh ginger, grated
- Salt and pepper to taste (use salt substitute if necessary)

Instructions:

1. Heat olive oil in a large skillet or wok over medium heat.
2. Add the chicken slices and cook for 5-6 minutes, until browned and cooked through.
3. Add the bell pepper, zucchini, garlic, and ginger to the skillet. Stir-fry for an additional 3-4 minutes.
4. Stir in the soy sauce, rice vinegar, sesame oil, salt, and pepper. Cook for 2 more minutes.
5. Serve hot.
6. Heat olive oil in a large skillet or wok over medium heat.
7. Add the chicken slices and cook for 5-6 minutes, until browned and cooked through.
8. Heat olive oil in a large skillet or wok over medium heat.
9. Add the chicken slices and cook for 5-6 minutes, until browned and cooked through.

Nutritional Information (per serving):

- Calories: 280
- Protein: 35g
- Carbs: 12g
- Fiber: 3g
- Potassium: 600mg
- Sodium: 220mg

Tip: For extra flavor, garnish with sesame seeds and sliced green onions.

Grilled Turkey Burgers with Sautéed Spinach

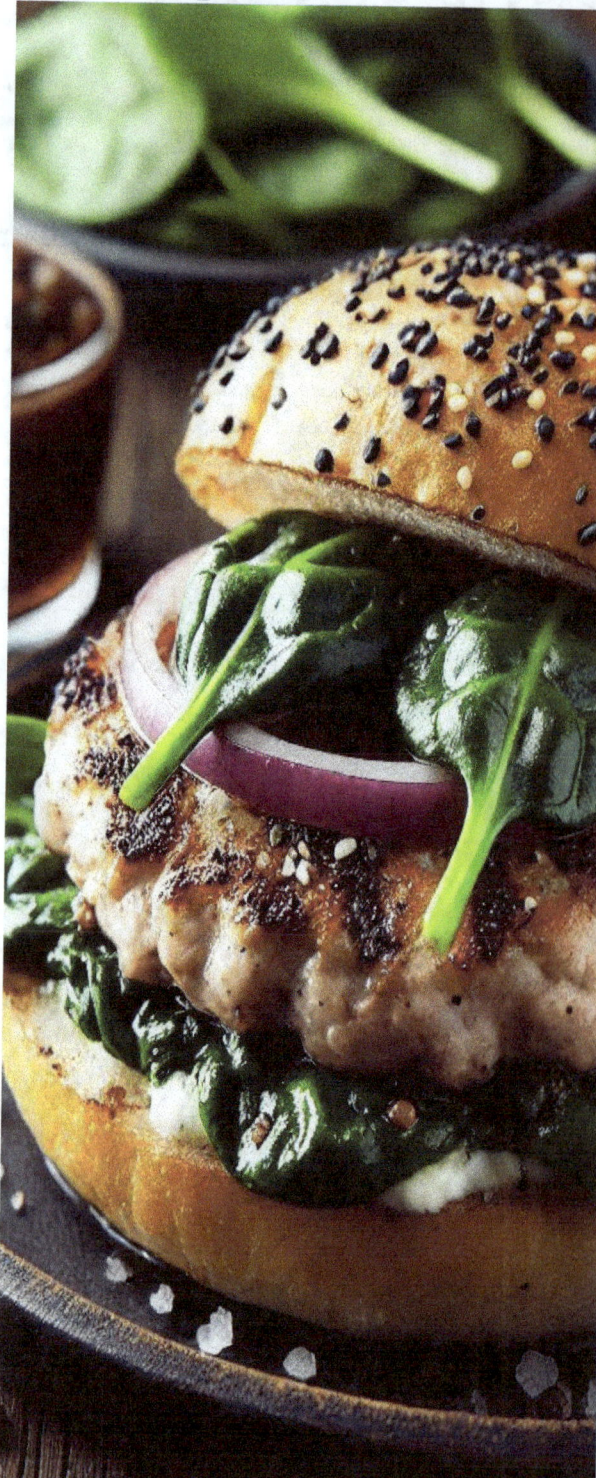

Prep Time: 10 minutes
Cooking Time: 15 minutes
Serves: 2
Ingredients:

- 1 pound ground turkey
- 1/4 cup finely chopped onion
- 1/2 teaspoon garlic powder
- 1/2 teaspoon dried oregano
- Salt and pepper to taste (use salt substitute if necessary)
- 2 cups fresh spinach, sautéed
- 1 tablespoon olive oil

Instructions:

1. Preheat the grill or grill pan over medium heat.
2. In a bowl, combine the ground turkey, onion, garlic powder, oregano, salt, and pepper. Form the mixture into two patties.
3. Grill the turkey burgers for 6-7 minutes on each side, until cooked through.
4. In a skillet, heat olive oil over medium heat and sauté the spinach until wilted, about 3-4 minutes.
5. Serve the burgers with sautéed spinach on the side.

Nutritional Information (per serving):

- Calories: 330
- Protein: 40g
- Carbs: 5g
- Fiber: 3g
- Potassium: 600mg
- Sodium: 170mg

Tip: For added flavor, top the turkey burgers with a small slice of low-sodium cheese.

Quinoa-Stuffed Eggplant

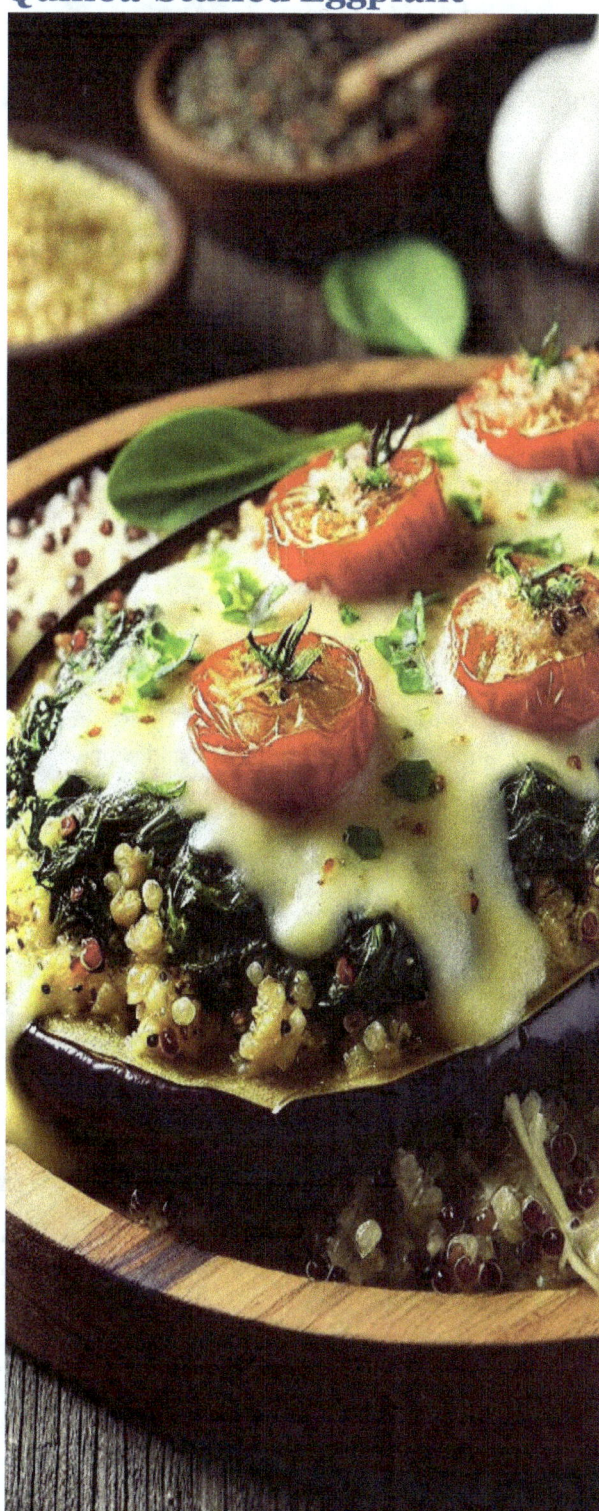

Prep Time: 15 minutes
Cooking Time: 40 minutes
Serves: 2
Ingredients:

- 1 large eggplant, halved and scooped out
- 1/2 cup cooked quinoa
- 1/4 cup diced tomatoes
- 1/4 cup onion, diced
- 1 tablespoon olive oil
- 1/2 teaspoon cumin
- Salt and pepper to taste (use salt substitute if necessary)

Instructions:

1. Preheat the oven to 375°F (190°C).
2. Drizzle the eggplant halves with olive oil, sprinkle with salt and pepper, and place on a baking sheet.
3. Roast the eggplant for 20 minutes until tender.
4. Meanwhile, heat olive oil in a skillet over medium heat. Add the onion and cook until soft, about 5 minutes.
5. Stir in the diced tomatoes, quinoa, cumin, salt, and pepper. Cook for another 5 minutes.
6. Stuff the roasted eggplant halves with the quinoa mixture.
7. Return to the oven and bake for an additional 10 minutes. Serve warm.

Nutritional Information (per serving):

- Calories: 280
- Protein: 8g
- Carbs: 38g
- Fiber: 10g
- Potassium: 750mg
- Sodium: 150mg

Tip: For extra richness, top the stuffed eggplant with a spoonful of low-fat Greek yogurt.

Baked Cod with Garlic and Roasted Brussels Sprouts

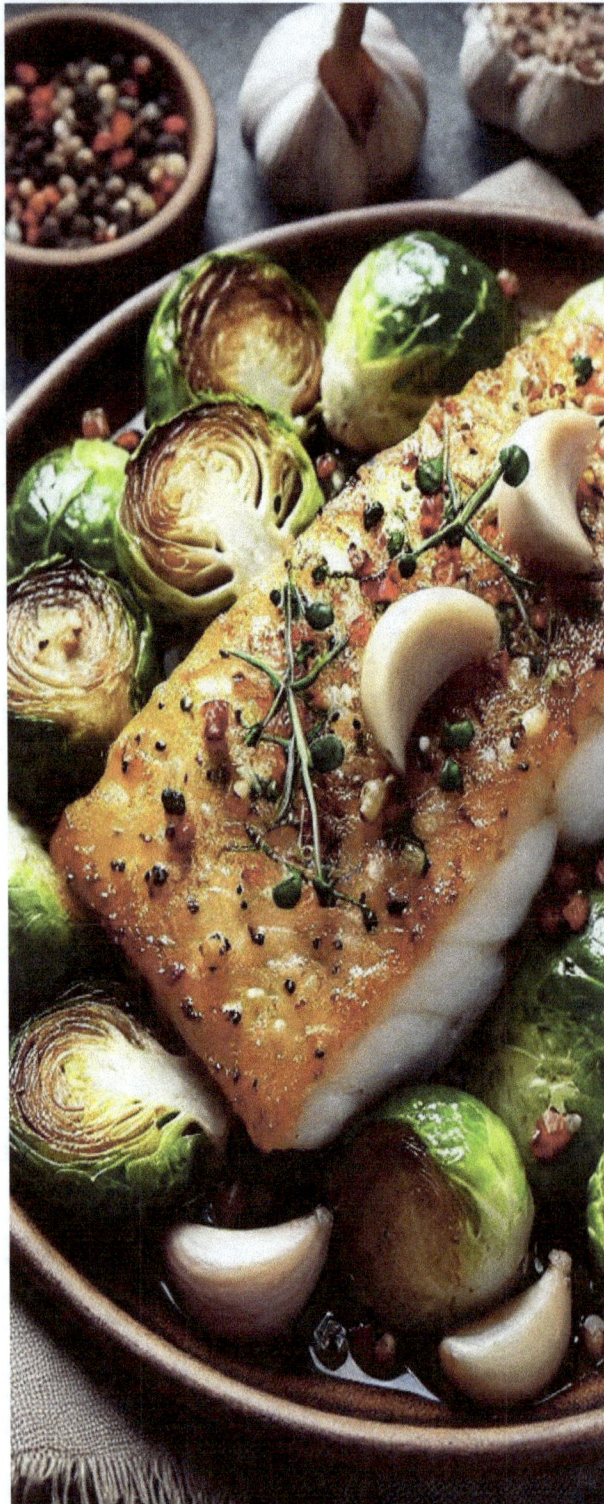

Prep Time: 10 minutes
Cooking Time: 25 minutes
Serves: 2
Ingredients:

- 2 cod fillets (4-6 oz each)
- 1 tablespoon olive oil
- 1 teaspoon garlic, minced
- 1 teaspoon lemon juice
- 1 cup Brussels sprouts, halved
- Salt and pepper to taste (use salt substitute if necessary)

Instructions:

1. Preheat the oven to 375°F (190°C).
2. Drizzle olive oil over the cod fillets, then sprinkle with garlic, lemon juice, salt, and pepper.
3. Arrange the Brussels sprouts on a baking sheet and drizzle with olive oil, salt, and pepper.
4. Bake the cod fillets for 15-20 minutes, or until cooked through.
5. Roast the Brussels sprouts for 20-25 minutes until crispy and tender.
6. Serve the cod fillets with roasted Brussels sprouts.

Nutritional Information (per serving):

- Calories: 320
- Protein: 35g
- Carbs: 15g
- Fiber: 5g
- Potassium: 700mg
- Sodium: 180mg

Tip: Serve with a drizzle of balsamic glaze over the Brussels sprouts for added flavor.

Low-Sodium Beef Stir Fry with Snow Peas

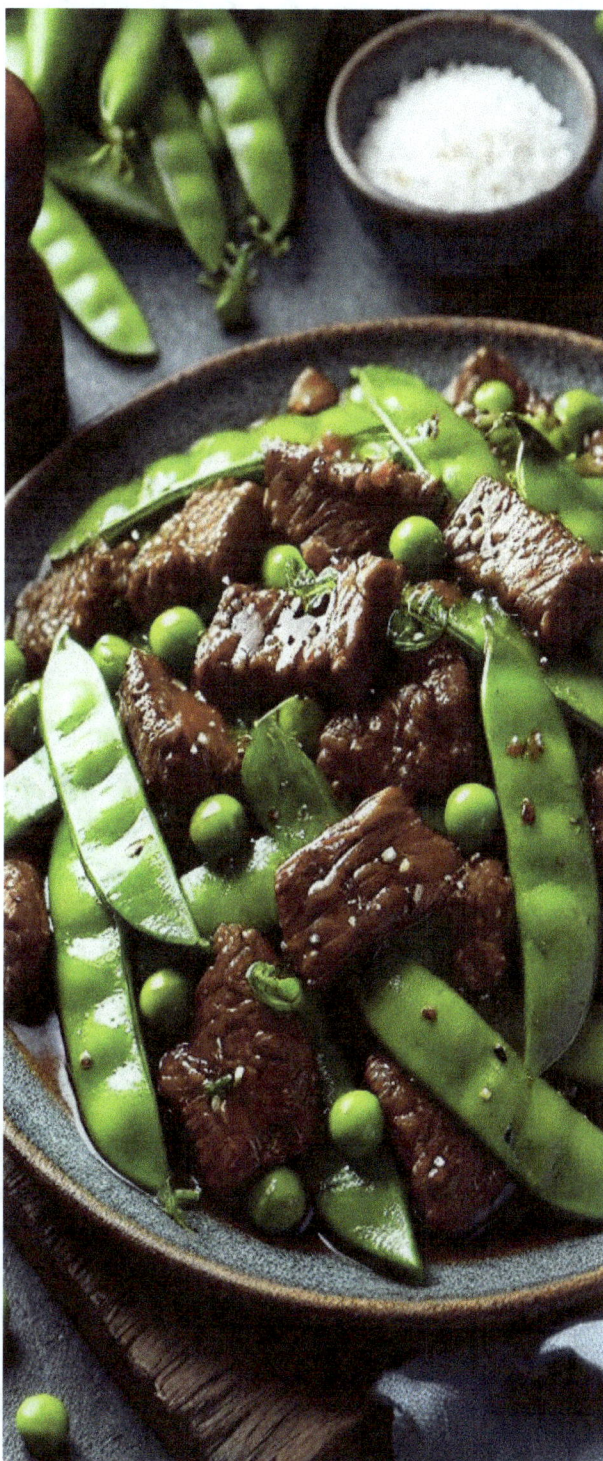

Prep Time: 15 minutes
Cooking Time: 10 minutes
Serves: 2
Ingredients:

- 1/2 pound lean beef, thinly sliced
- 1 cup snow peas
- 1/4 cup low-sodium soy sauce
- 1 tablespoon sesame oil
- 1 teaspoon garlic, minced
- 1 teaspoon fresh ginger, grated
- 1 tablespoon rice vinegar
- 1 tablespoon green onions, chopped

Instructions:

1. Heat sesame oil in a skillet or wok over medium-high heat.
2. Add the beef and cook for 5-6 minutes, until browned.
3. Stir in the garlic, ginger, snow peas, soy sauce, and rice vinegar. Cook for an additional 3-4 minutes until the snow peas are tender but still crisp.
4. Serve the stir-fry hot, garnished with chopped green onions.

Nutritional Information (per serving):

- Calories: 300
- Protein: 35g
- Carbs: 12g
- Fiber: 4g
- Potassium: 500mg
- Sodium: 250mg

Tip: Serve with brown rice or quinoa to make this a more filling meal.

Chicken and Sweet Potato Mash

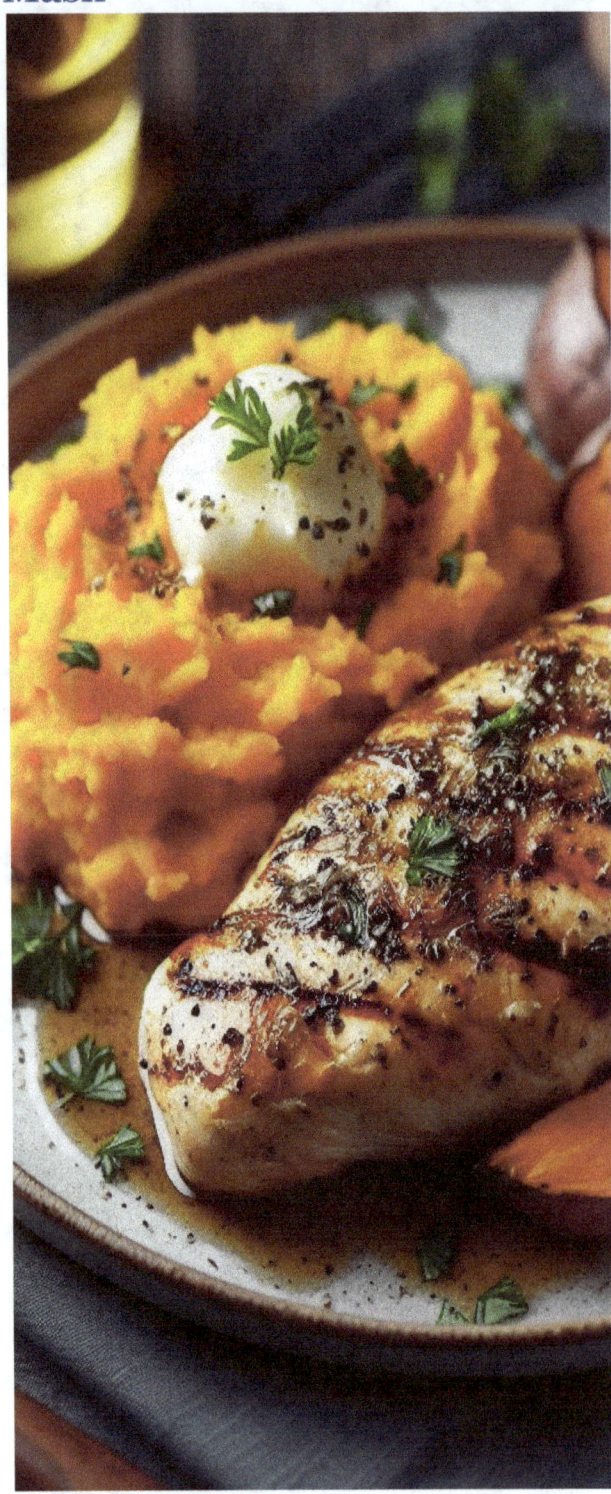

Prep Time: 15 minutes
Cooking Time: 30 minutes
Serves: 2
Ingredients:

- 2 chicken breasts
- 2 medium sweet potatoes, peeled and cubed
- 1 tablespoon olive oil
- 1/2 teaspoon cinnamon
- Salt and pepper to taste (use salt substitute if necessary)

Instructions:

1. Preheat the oven to 375°F (190°C).
2. Roast the sweet potatoes in olive oil, cinnamon, salt, and pepper for 20-25 minutes or until soft.
3. Meanwhile, pan-sear the chicken breasts in olive oil over medium heat for 6-7 minutes per side, until fully cooked.
4. Mash the sweet potatoes and serve them alongside the chicken.

Nutritional Information (per serving):

- Calories: 350
- Protein: 35g
- Carbs: 32g
- Fiber: 5g
- Potassium: 800mg
- Sodium: 150mg

Tip: Add a sprinkle of nutmeg for extra warmth in the mashed sweet potatoes.

Vegetarian Lentil Stew

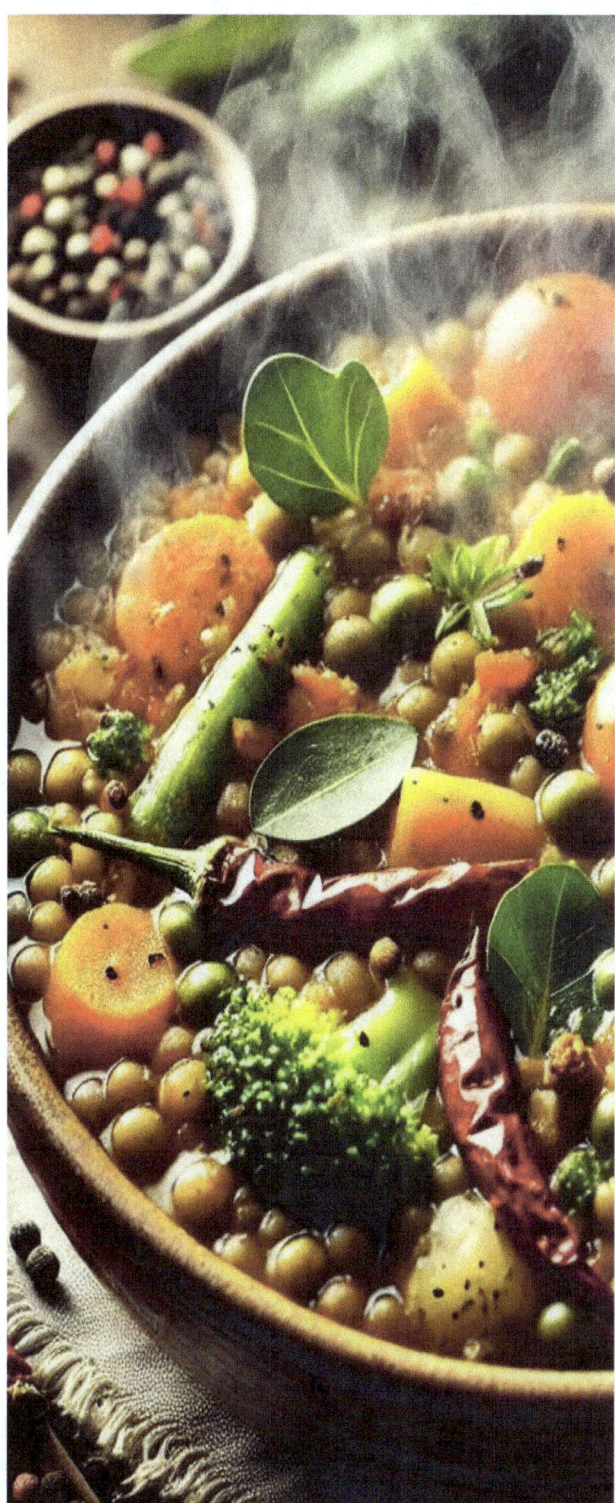

Prep Time: 15 minutes
Cooking Time: 45 minutes
Serves: 4
Ingredients:

- 1 cup dried lentils, rinsed
- 1 tablespoon olive oil
- 1 onion, chopped
- 2 carrots, diced
- 2 celery stalks, diced
- 1 zucchini, diced
- 2 cloves garlic, minced
- 1 teaspoon ground cumin
- 1/2 teaspoon turmeric
- 1/2 teaspoon dried thyme
- 4 cups low-sodium vegetable broth
- 1 cup diced tomatoes
- Salt and pepper to taste (use salt substitute if necessary)

Instructions:

- In a large pot, heat olive oil over medium heat.
- Add the onion, carrots, and celery, cooking for 5 minutes until softened.
- Stir in the garlic, cumin, turmeric, and thyme, cooking for another 1-2 minutes.
- Add the lentils, vegetable broth, diced tomatoes, zucchini, salt, and pepper. Bring to a boil.
- Lower the heat and simmer for 35-40 minutes, or until the lentils are tender.
- Serve the stew hot with a side of whole-grain bread.

Nutritional Information (per serving):

- Calories: 230
- Protein: 13g
- Carbs: 40g
- Fiber: 14g
- Potassium: 650mg
- Sodium: 180mg

Tip: For extra creaminess, stir in a spoonful of plain Greek yogurt just before serving.

Turkey Meatballs with Zucchini Noodles

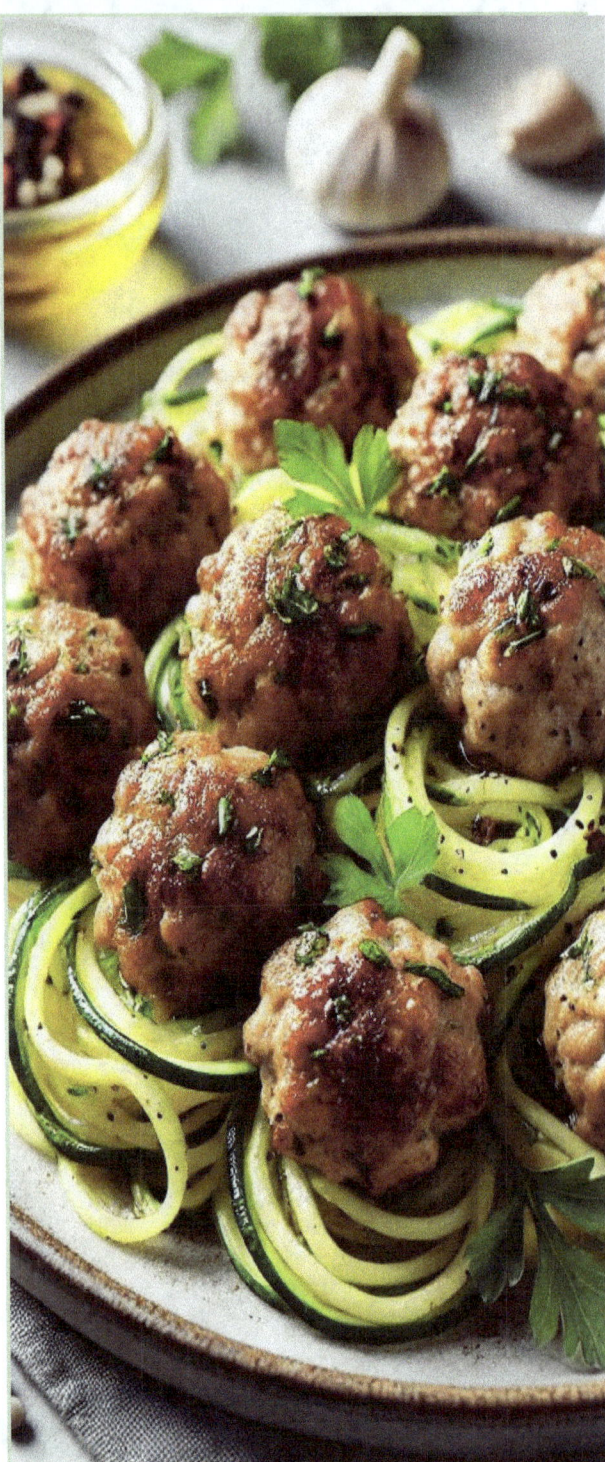

Prep Time: 20 minutes
Cooking Time: 25 minutes

Serves: 2

Ingredients:

- 1/2 pound lean ground turkey
- 1/4 cup whole-wheat breadcrumbs
- 1/4 cup grated Parmesan (optional, low-sodium)
- 1 egg
- 1 teaspoon garlic powder
- 1 teaspoon dried basil
- 1 teaspoon dried oregano
- Salt and pepper to taste (use salt substitute if necessary)
- 2 medium zucchinis, spiralized into noodles
- 1 tablespoon olive oil
- 1/2 cup low-sodium marinara sauce

Instructions:

- Preheat the oven to 375°F (190°C).
- In a bowl, mix the ground turkey, breadcrumbs, Parmesan, egg, garlic powder, basil, oregano, salt, and pepper. Form the mixture into 12-14 small meatballs.
- Place the meatballs on a baking sheet and bake for 20 minutes, or until cooked through.
- While the meatballs bake, heat olive oil in a skillet over medium heat. Add the zucchini noodles and sauté for 2-3 minutes, just until tender.
- Heat the marinara sauce in a separate pan.
- Serve the meatballs on top of the zucchini noodles, topped with the marinara sauce.

Nutritional Information (per serving):

- Calories: 350
- Protein: 40g
- Carbs: 18g
- Fiber: 6g
- Potassium: 800mg
- Sodium: 220mg

Tip: If you prefer a firmer texture, sauté the zucchini noodles for a shorter time to maintain their crunch.

Roast Chicken with Carrots and Potatoes

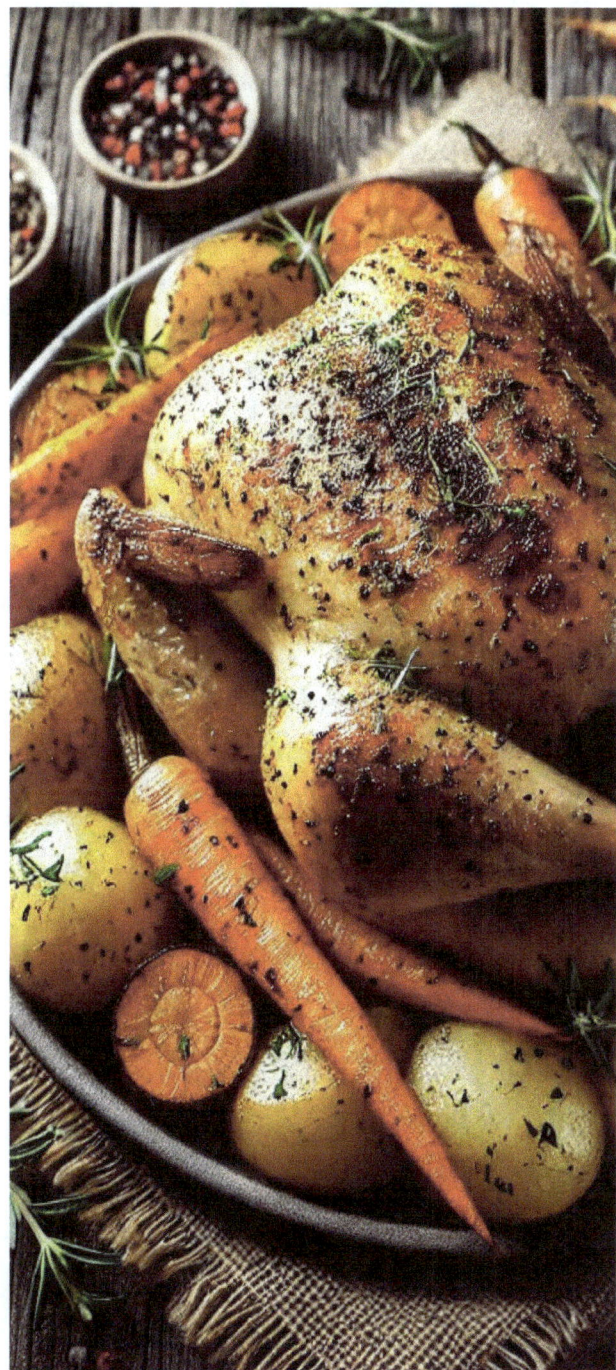

Prep Time: 15 minutes
Cooking Time: 60 minutes
Serves: 4

Ingredients:

- 4 bone-in, skin-on chicken thighs
- 4 medium potatoes, diced
- 4 large carrots, peeled and cut into chunks
- 2 tablespoons olive oil
- 1 teaspoon dried rosemary
- 1 teaspoon garlic powder
- Salt and pepper to taste (use salt substitute if necessary)

Instructions:

1. Preheat the oven to 400°F (200°C).
2. Arrange the chicken thighs on a baking sheet. Drizzle with olive oil and sprinkle with rosemary, garlic powder, salt, and pepper.
3. Add the diced potatoes and carrots to the baking sheet, tossing with a bit of olive oil, salt, and pepper.
4. Roast for 50-60 minutes, or until the chicken is golden and the potatoes and carrots are tender.
5. Serve hot.

Nutritional Information (per serving):

- Calories: 420
- Protein: 35g
- Carbs: 30g
- Fiber: 6g
- Potassium: 950mg
- Sodium: 220mg

Tip: For extra flavor, rub the chicken with fresh lemon zest and thyme before roasting.

Grilled Shrimp with Cilantro-Lime Quinoa

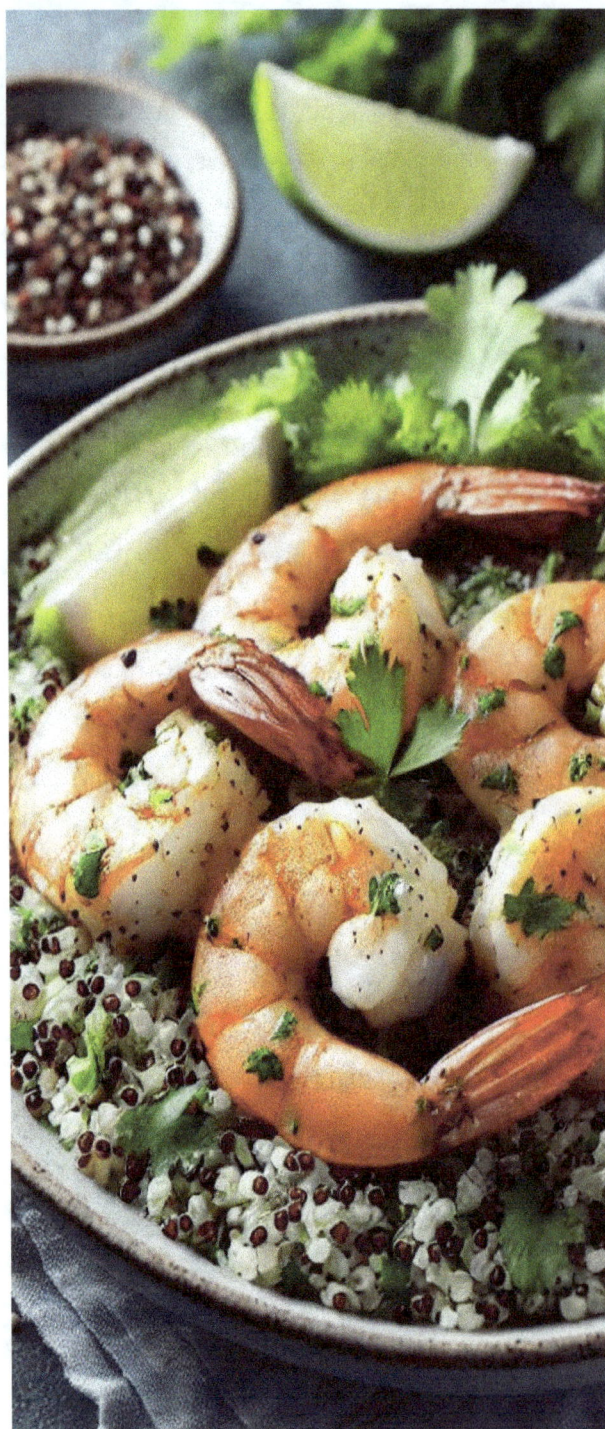

Prep Time: 15 minutes

Cooking Time: 10 minutes

Serves: 2

Ingredients:

- 1/2 pound large shrimp, peeled and deveined
- 1 tablespoon olive oil
- 1 tablespoon lime juice
- 1/2 teaspoon chili powder
- Salt and pepper to taste (use salt substitute if necessary)
- 1 cup cooked quinoa
- 1/4 cup fresh cilantro, chopped
- 1 tablespoon lime juice (for quinoa)

Instructions:

1. Preheat the grill to medium-high heat.
2. Toss the shrimp with olive oil, lime juice, chili powder, salt, and pepper.
3. Grill the shrimp for 2-3 minutes per side, until pink and opaque.
4. Meanwhile, mix the cooked quinoa with chopped cilantro and lime juice.
5. Serve the shrimp over a bed of cilantro-lime quinoa.

Nutritional Information (per serving):

- Calories: 350
- Protein: 30g
- Carbs: 32g
- Fiber: 5g
- Potassium: 550mg
- Sodium: 230mg

Tip: For added crunch, garnish with toasted pumpkin seeds or crushed almonds.

Baked Tofu with Steamed Broccoli and Brown Rice

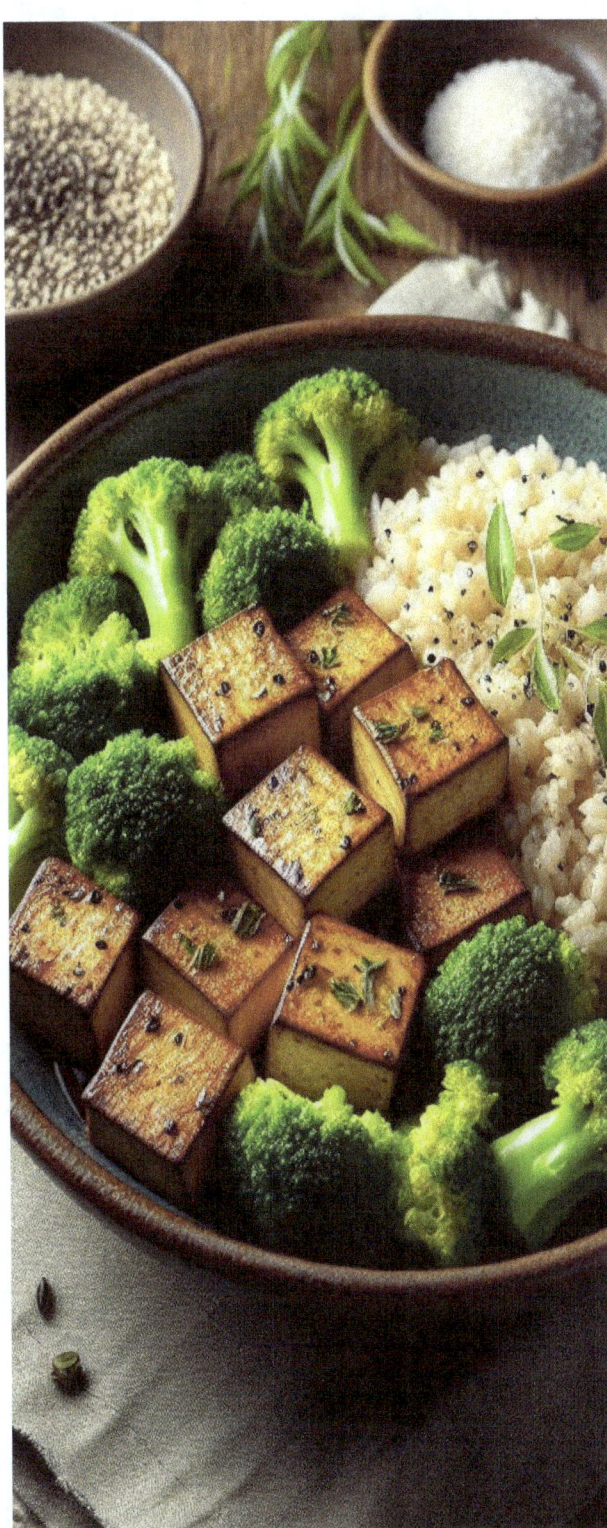

Prep Time: 15 minutes
Cooking Time: 30 minutes
Serves: 2

Ingredients:

- 1 block firm tofu, pressed and cubed
- 1 tablespoon soy sauce (low-sodium)
- 1 teaspoon sesame oil
- 1 tablespoon olive oil
- 2 cups broccoli florets
- 1 cup cooked brown rice

Instructions:

1. Preheat the oven to 375°F (190°C).
2. Toss the tofu cubes with soy sauce, sesame oil, and olive oil.
3. Spread the tofu on a baking sheet and bake for 25-30 minutes, flipping halfway through.
4. Steam the broccoli florets for 5-6 minutes until tender.
5. Serve the tofu over brown rice, with steamed broccoli on the side.

Nutritional Information (per serving):

- Calories: 350
- Protein: 20g
- Carbs: 40g
- Fiber: 8g
- Potassium: 800mg
- Sodium: 200mg

Tip: For extra flavor, drizzle the tofu with a bit of balsamic vinegar or low-sodium teriyaki sauce before serving.

Stuffed Portobello Mushrooms with Quinoa and Spinach

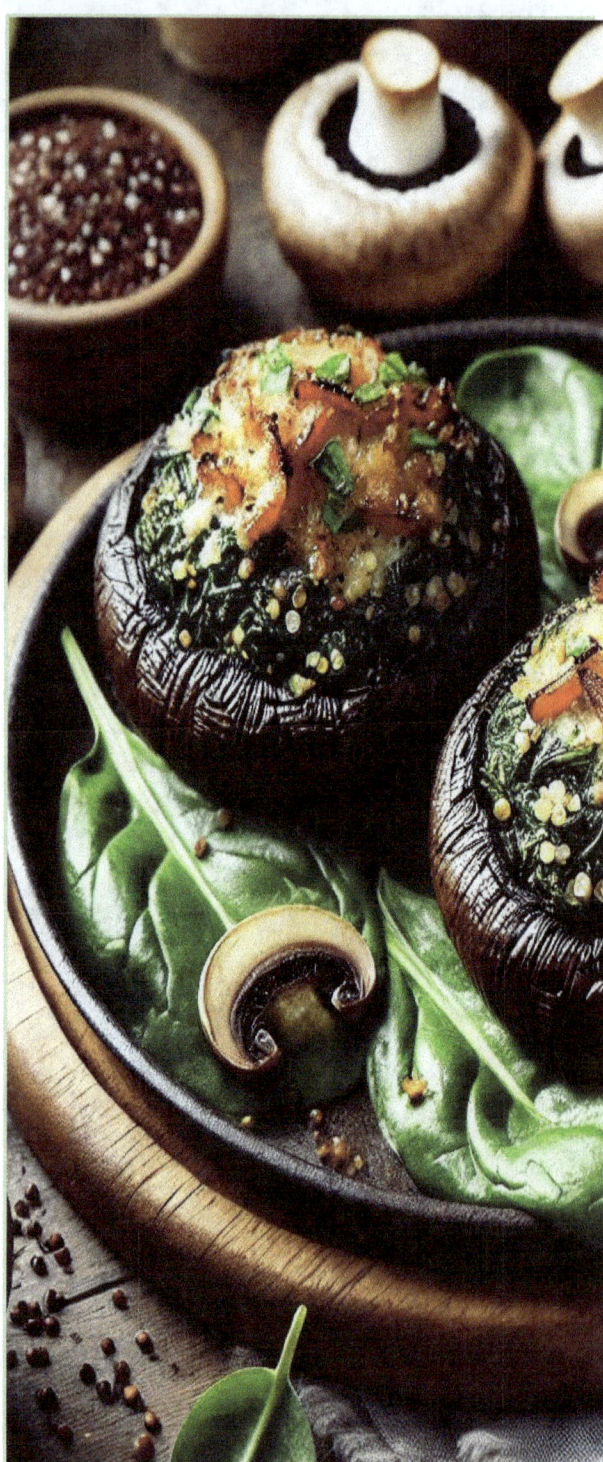

Prep Time: 10 minutes

Cooking Time: 25 minutes

Serves: 2

Ingredients:

- 2 large Portobello mushroom caps
- 1/2 cup cooked quinoa
- 1 cup spinach, chopped
- 1/4 cup low-sodium feta cheese (optional)
- 1 tablespoon olive oil
- 1 teaspoon garlic powder
- Salt and pepper to taste (use salt substitute if necessary)

Instructions:

1. Preheat the oven to 375°F (190°C).
2. Remove the stems from the mushrooms and scoop out the gills.
3. In a bowl, combine quinoa, spinach, feta cheese, garlic powder, salt, and pepper.
4. Stuff the mushroom caps with the quinoa mixture.
5. Drizzle the stuffed mushrooms with olive oil and bake for 20-25 minutes until tender.
6. Serve immediately.

Nutritional Information (per serving):

- Calories: 280
- Protein: 12g
- Carbs: 35g
- Fiber: 7g
- Potassium: 600mg
- Sodium: 250mg

Tip: For an extra savory touch, top the stuffed mushrooms with a sprinkle of Parmesan before baking.

Cauliflower Crust Pizza with Low-Sodium Toppings

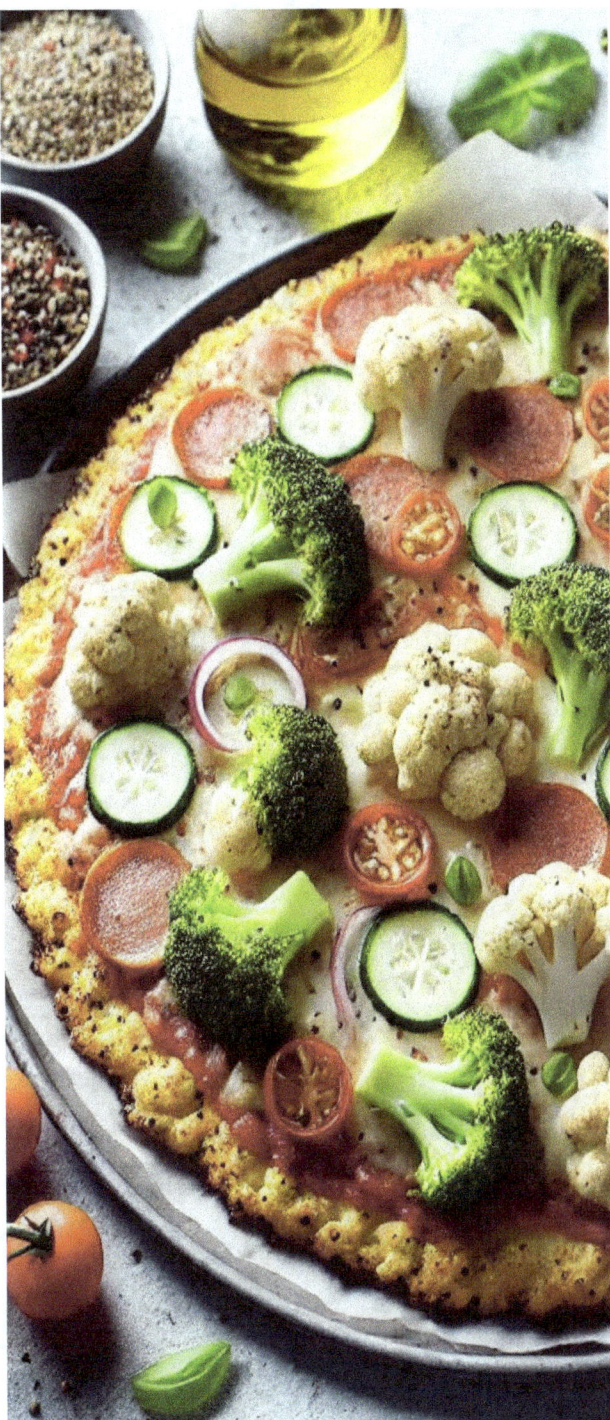

Prep Time: 15 minutes
Cooking Time: 30 minutes
Serves: 2

Ingredients:

- 1 medium cauliflower, grated
- 1 egg
- 1/4 cup shredded mozzarella cheese (optional)
- 1/2 teaspoon dried oregano
- 1/4 teaspoon garlic powder
- Salt and pepper to taste (use salt substitute if necessary)
- 1/4 cup low-sodium tomato sauce
- 1/4 cup bell peppers, diced
- 1/4 cup mushrooms, sliced

Instructions:

1. Preheat the oven to 400°F (200°C).
2. In a bowl, combine the grated cauliflower, egg, mozzarella, oregano, garlic powder, salt, and pepper.
3. Spread the mixture onto a baking sheet lined with parchment paper and bake for 20 minutes.
4. Remove from the oven, spread the tomato sauce on the crust, and top with bell peppers and mushrooms.
5. Bake for an additional 10 minutes, until the toppings are cooked and the crust is golden.
6. Serve hot.

Nutritional Information (per serving):

- Calories: 220
- Protein: 12g
- Carbs: 18g
- Fiber: 6g
- Potassium: 450mg
- Sodium: 180mg

Tip: Add a sprinkle of low-sodium Parmesan cheese for extra flavor.

Eggplant Parmesan (Kidney-Friendly Version)

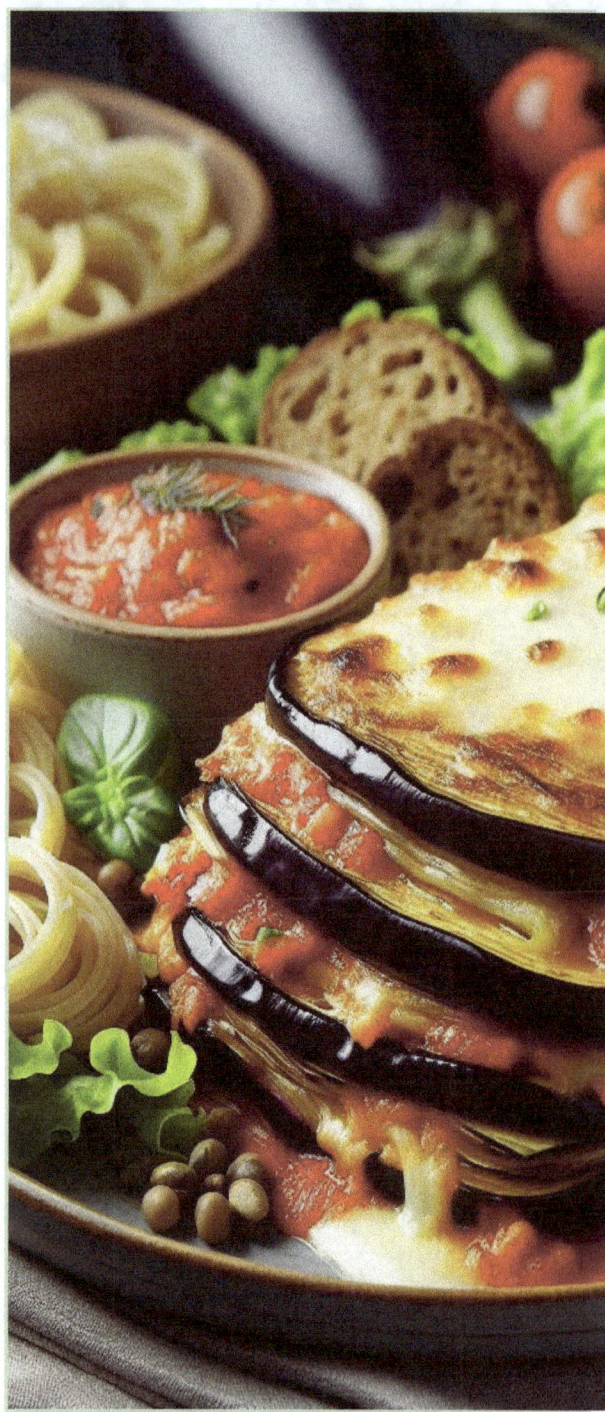

Prep Time: 20 minutes
Cooking Time: 40 minutes
Serves: 4

Ingredients:

- 1 large eggplant, sliced into rounds
- 1 cup whole-wheat breadcrumbs
- 1/2 cup low-sodium marinara sauce
- 1/4 cup low-sodium mozzarella cheese, shredded
- 1 tablespoon olive oil
- Salt and pepper to taste (use salt substitute if necessary)

Instructions:

1. Preheat the oven to 375°F (190°C).
2. Lightly coat the eggplant slices in olive oil and season with salt and pepper.
3. Dip each slice in breadcrumbs and place on a baking sheet. Bake for 25 minutes, flipping halfway through.
4. After baking, top each slice with marinara sauce and mozzarella cheese. Bake for another 10 minutes, or until the cheese melts.
5. Serve warm with a side of steamed vegetables.

Nutritional Information (per serving):

- Calories: 180
- Protein: 8g
- Carbs: 28g
- Fiber: 7g
- Potassium: 600mg
- Sodium: 210mg

Tip: For an extra crisp, bake the eggplant at a higher temperature for the first few minutes.

Chapter 6

Desserts

Banana-Free Chocolate Avocado Mousse

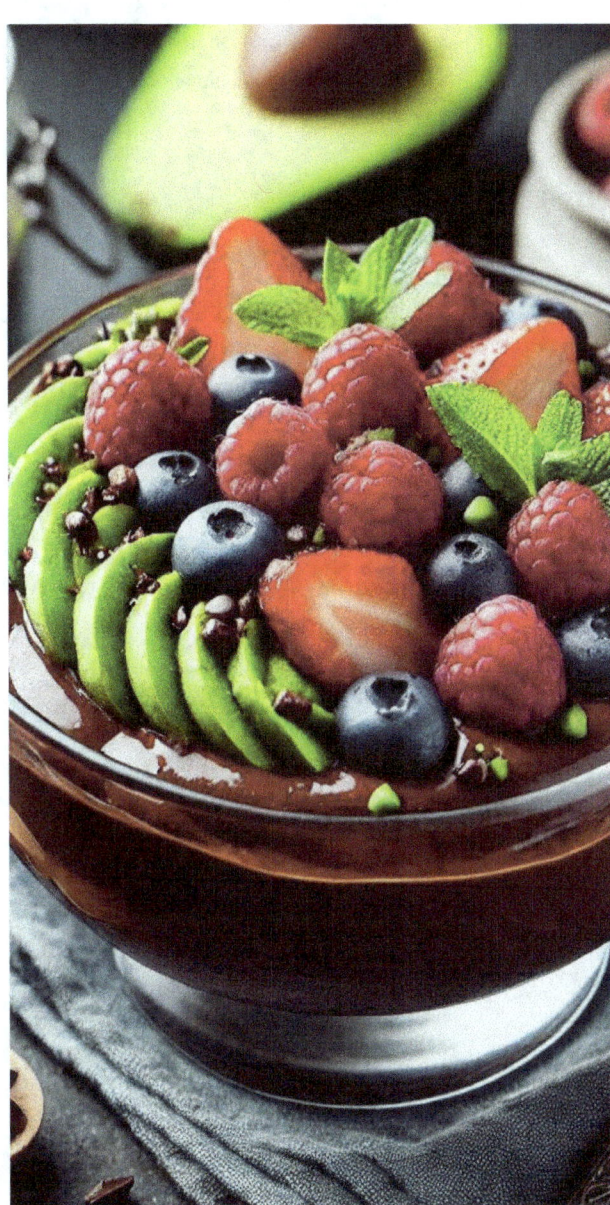

Prep Time: 10 minutes
Cooking Time: 0 minutes

Serves: 4
Ingredients:

- 2 ripe avocados, peeled and pitted
- 1/4 cup unsweetened cocoa powder
- 1/4 cup maple syrup or honey
- 1 teaspoon vanilla extract
- 1/4 cup almond milk (or preferred milk alternative)
- Pinch of sea salt

Instructions:

- In a blender or food processor, combine the avocados, cocoa powder, maple syrup, vanilla, almond milk, and sea salt.
- Blend until smooth and creamy.
- Taste and adjust sweetness by adding more maple syrup if necessary.
- Spoon the mousse into serving bowls and refrigerate for at least 1 hour before serving.
- Garnish with a sprinkle of cocoa powder or fresh berries, if desired.

Nutritional Information (per serving):

- Calories: 160
- Protein: 2g
- Carbs: 15g
- Fiber: 7g
- Potassium: 450mg
- Sodium: 10mg

Tip: For a richer flavor, use coconut milk instead of almond milk.

Apple Crisp with Oats and Cinnamon

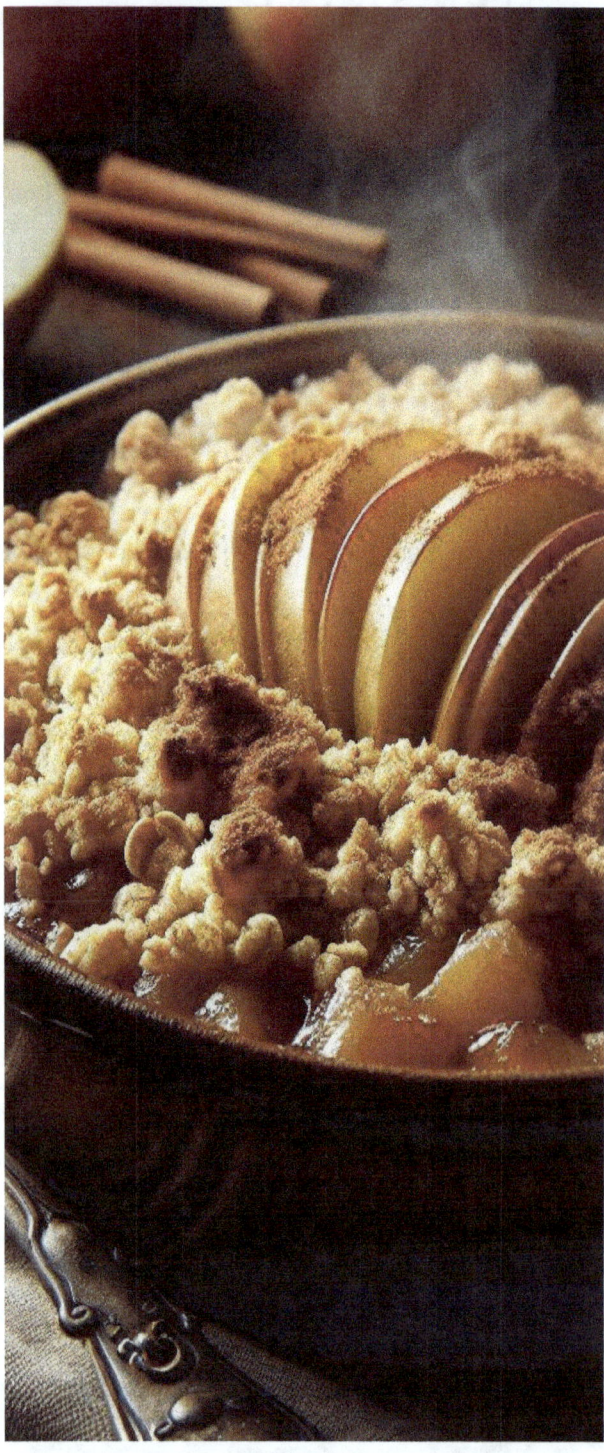

Prep Time: 15 minutes
Cooking Time: 45 minutes

Serves: 6
Ingredients:

- 4 large apples, peeled, cored, and sliced
- 1/2 teaspoon cinnamon
- 1/4 cup rolled oats
- 2 tablespoons almond flour
- 2 tablespoons coconut sugar
- 1/4 cup coconut oil, melted
- 1/2 teaspoon vanilla extract
- Pinch of salt

Instructions:

- Preheat the oven to 350°F (175°C).
- Toss the apple slices with cinnamon in a baking dish.
- In a bowl, combine oats, almond flour, coconut sugar, melted coconut oil, vanilla extract, and a pinch of salt.
- Sprinkle the oat mixture over the apples.
- Bake for 40-45 minutes, until the apples are tender and the top is golden brown.
- Serve warm, optionally with a scoop of low-sodium vanilla yogurt.

Nutritional Information (per serving):

- Calories: 180
- Protein: 2g
- Carbs: 24g
- Fiber: 5g
- Potassium: 350mg
- Sodium: 10mg

Tip: To make this recipe even more kidney-friendly, replace coconut sugar with a natural sweetener like stevia or monk fruit.

Homemade Coconut Milk Popsicles

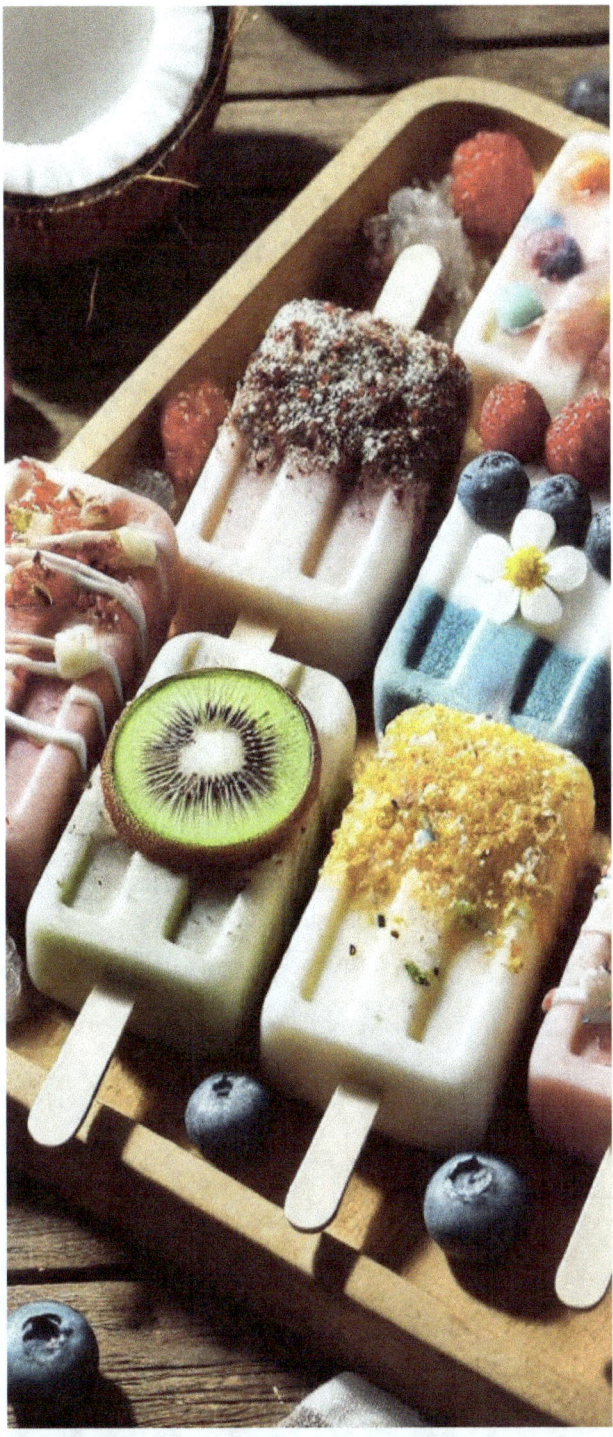

Prep Time: 10 minutes
Cooking Time: 0 minutes

Serves: 6

Ingredients:

- 1 can (13.5 oz) full-fat coconut milk
- 1 tablespoon honey or maple syrup
- 1/2 teaspoon vanilla extract
- 1/4 cup unsweetened shredded coconut
- 1/4 cup fresh berries (optional)

Instructions:

- In a bowl, whisk together the coconut milk, honey, and vanilla extract until well combined.
- Pour the mixture into popsicle molds, filling each mold about 3/4 full.
- Sprinkle shredded coconut and a few fresh berries into each mold.
- Insert sticks and freeze for at least 4 hours or until completely set.
- To release the popsicles, run warm water over the outside of the mold for a few seconds.

Nutritional Information (per serving):

- Calories: 130
- Protein: 1g
- Carbs: 8g
- Fiber: 2g
- Potassium: 160mg
- Sodium: 5mg

Tip: For added variety, blend in some fresh mango or strawberry puree before freezing.

Low-Sodium Almond Butter Cookies

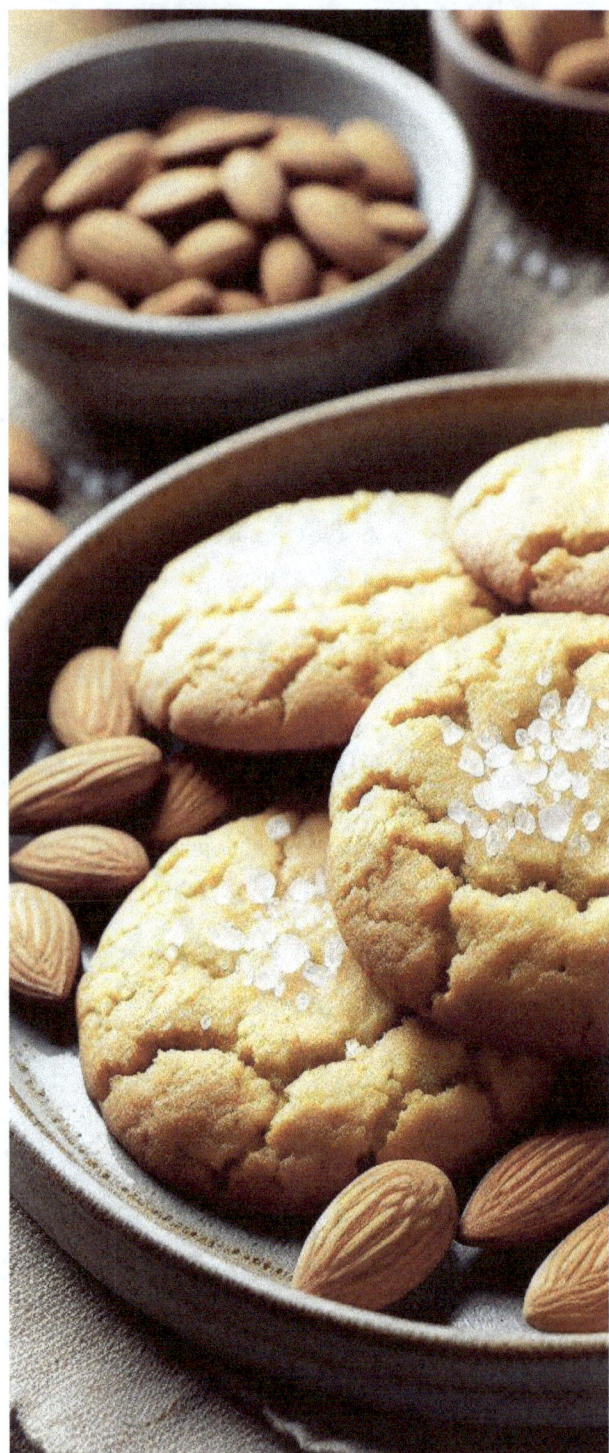

Prep Time: 10 minutes
Cooking Time: 12 minutes
Serves: 12
Ingredients:

- 1 cup almond butter
- 1/4 cup coconut sugar
- 1 egg
- 1 teaspoon vanilla extract
- 1/4 teaspoon baking soda
- 1/4 teaspoon cinnamon
- Pinch of salt

Instructions:

- Preheat the oven to 350°F (175°C).
- In a bowl, mix together the almond butter, coconut sugar, egg, vanilla extract, baking soda, cinnamon, and a pinch of salt.
- Scoop tablespoon-sized portions of dough and roll into balls. Place them on a baking sheet lined with parchment paper.
- Flatten each dough ball with a fork.
- Bake for 10-12 minutes, until the cookies are golden brown.
- Let the cookies cool completely before serving.

Nutritional Information (per serving):

- Calories: 110
- Protein: 3g
- Carbs: 6g
- Fiber: 2g
- Potassium: 150mg
- Sodium: 10mg

Tip: For extra flavor, add a handful of dark chocolate chips or chopped walnuts to the dough before baking.

Berry Sorbet with a Touch of Lime

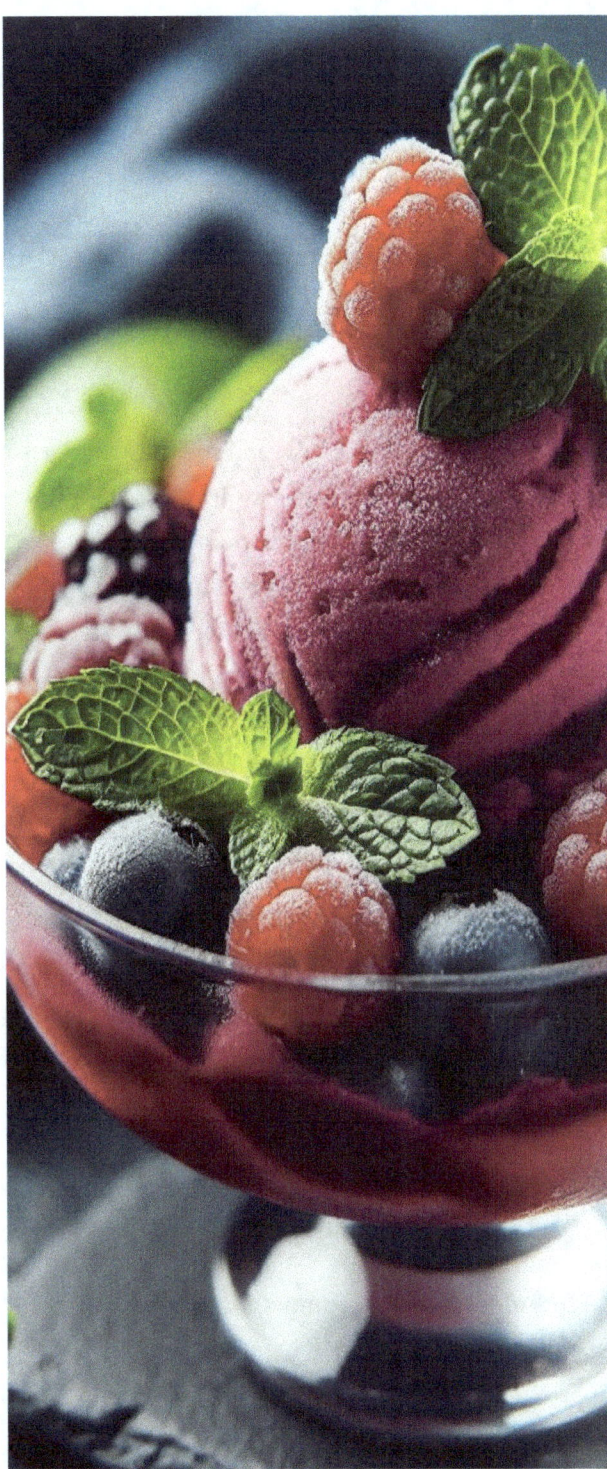

Prep Time: 10 minutes

Cooking Time: 0 minutes

Serves: 4

Ingredients:

- 2 cups mixed berries (strawberries, raspberries, blueberries, etc.)
- 1/4 cup fresh lime juice
- 1 tablespoon honey or agave syrup
- 1/4 cup water

Instructions:

- In a blender, combine the berries, lime juice, honey, and water.
- Blend until smooth, then taste and adjust sweetness as needed.
- Pour the mixture into a shallow dish and freeze for about 2 hours.
- Once frozen, scrape the sorbet with a fork to create a fluffy texture.
- Serve immediately for a refreshing treat.

Nutritional Information (per serving):

- Calories: 70
- Protein: 1g
- Carbs: 17g
- Fiber: 4g
- Potassium: 250mg
- Sodium: 5mg

Tip: For a smoother texture, use a food processor instead of a blender and freeze overnight.

Chia Seed Pudding with Cacao and Almond Butter

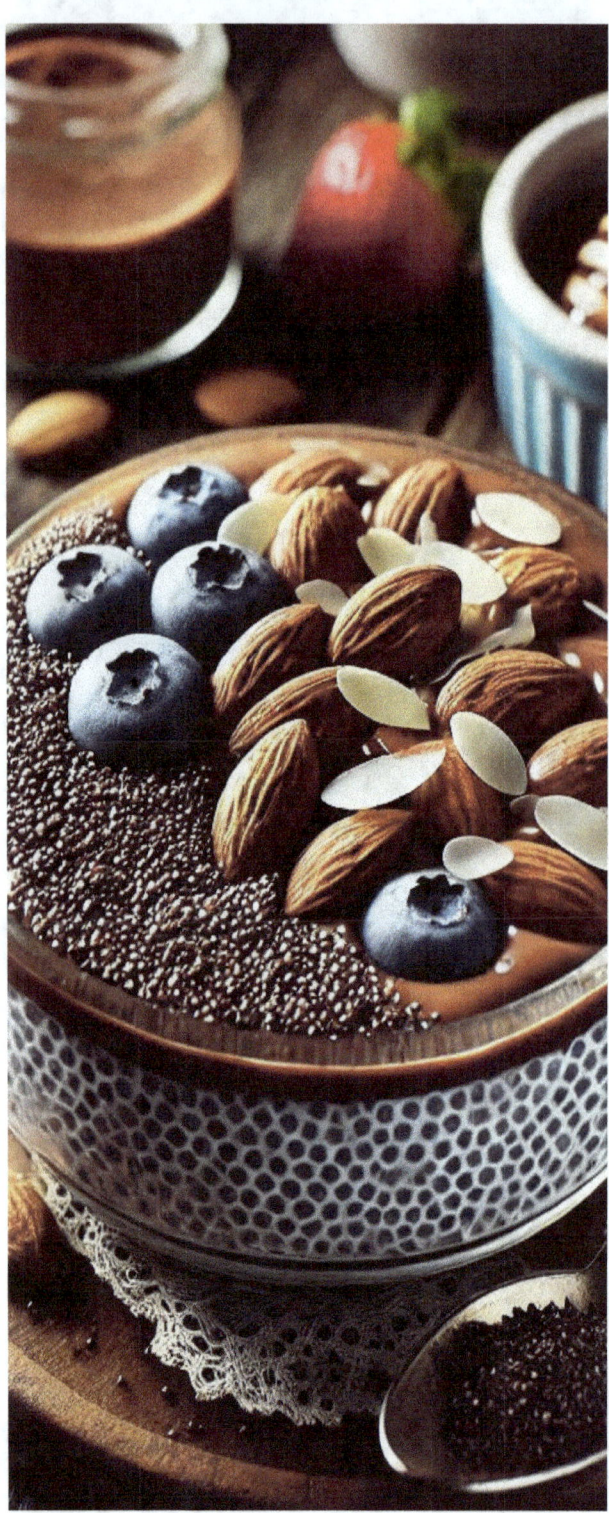

Prep Time: 5 minutes
Cooking Time: 0 minutes
Serves: 2
Ingredients:

- 2 tablespoons chia seeds
- 1 cup unsweetened almond milk
- 1 tablespoon cacao powder
- 1 tablespoon almond butter
- 1 teaspoon maple syrup

Instructions:

- In a bowl, combine the chia seeds, almond milk, cacao powder, almond butter, and maple syrup.
- Stir well to combine, then cover and refrigerate for at least 2 hours or overnight to allow the chia seeds to thicken.
- Stir the pudding before serving, and top with fresh berries or sliced almonds.

Nutritional Information (per serving):

- Calories: 210
- Protein: 6g
- Carbs: 16g
- Fiber: 9g
- Potassium: 150mg
- Sodium: 5mg

Tip: Add a sprinkle of cinnamon or a dash of vanilla extract for extra flavor.

Carrot Cake Energy Balls

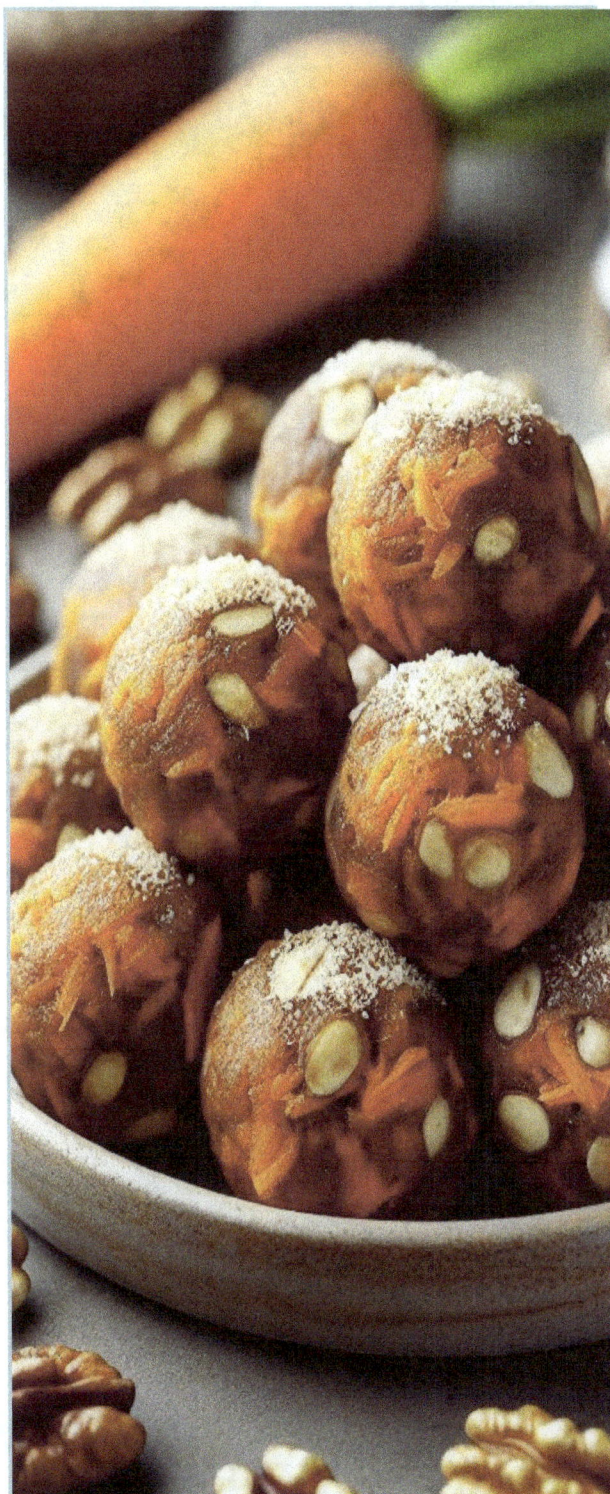

Prep Time: 15 minutes
Cooking Time: 0 minutes

Serves: 12
Ingredients:

- 1 cup rolled oats
- 1/2 cup unsweetened shredded coconut
- 1/2 cup grated carrots
- 1/4 cup almond flour
- 1 tablespoon chia seeds
- 2 tablespoons honey
- 1 teaspoon cinnamon
- Pinch of salt

Instructions:

- In a food processor, combine the oats, shredded coconut, grated carrots, almond flour, chia seeds, honey, cinnamon, and salt.
- Pulse until everything is well combined and the mixture starts to stick together.
- Roll the mixture into small balls (about 1 inch in diameter).
- Refrigerate the energy balls for at least 30 minutes before serving.

Nutritional Information (per serving):

- Calories: 120
- Protein: 3g
- Carbs: 18g
- Fiber: 4g
- Potassium: 220mg
- Sodium: 5mg

Tip: For extra sweetness, add a few chopped dates to the mixture before rolling into balls.

Baked Pears with Cinnamon and Walnuts

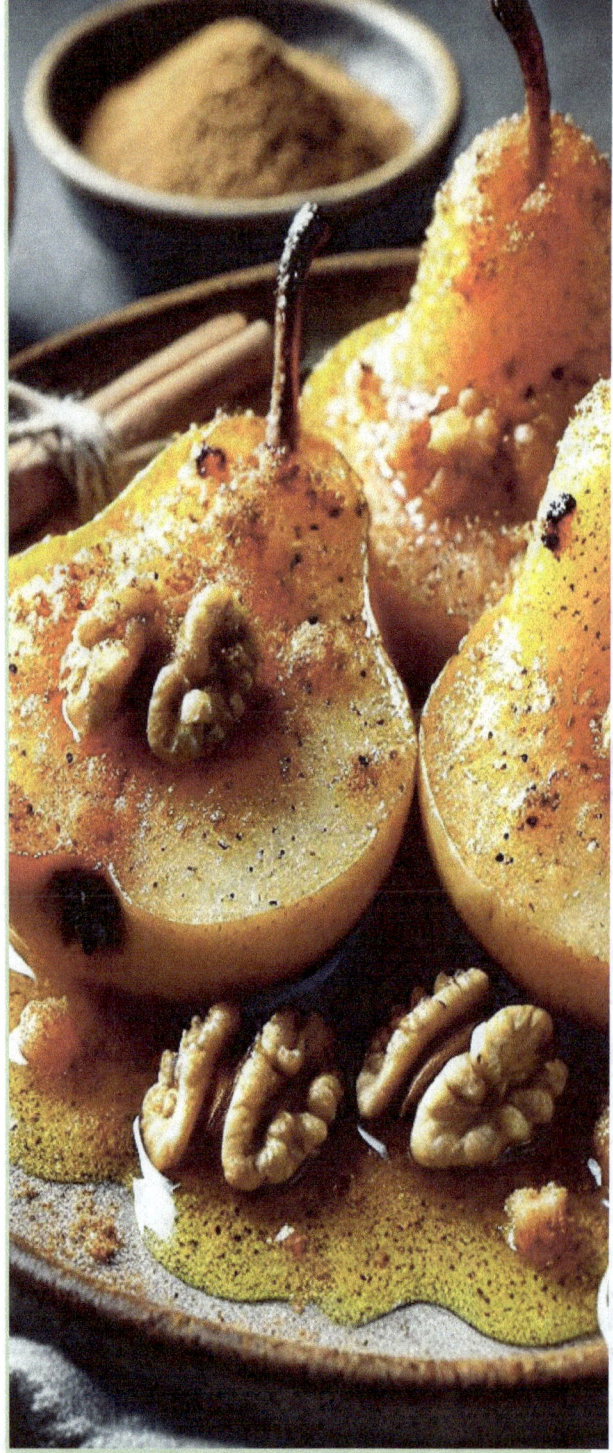

Prep Time: 10 minutes
Cooking Time: 25 minutes

Serves: 4

Ingredients:

- 4 ripe pears, halved and cored
- 1/4 cup chopped walnuts
- 1 teaspoon ground cinnamon
- 2 tablespoons honey or maple syrup
- 1/4 teaspoon vanilla extract
- 1 tablespoon lemon juice

Instructions:

- Preheat the oven to 350°F (175°C).
- Place the pear halves on a baking sheet lined with parchment paper.
- In a small bowl, mix together the walnuts, cinnamon, honey, vanilla, and lemon juice.
- Spoon the walnut mixture into the center of each pear half.
- Bake for 20-25 minutes, until the pears are tender and the topping is golden.
- Serve warm, optionally with a dollop of low-sodium whipped cream or Greek yogurt.

Nutritional Information (per serving):

- Calories: 170
- Protein: 3g
- Carbs: 30g
- Fiber: 6g
- Potassium: 250mg
- Sodium: 5mg

Tip: For added flavor, drizzle with a little more honey or a sprinkle of cinnamon before serving.

Gluten-Free Blueberry Muffins

Prep Time: 15 minutes
Cooking Time: 25 minutes
Serves: 6
Ingredients:

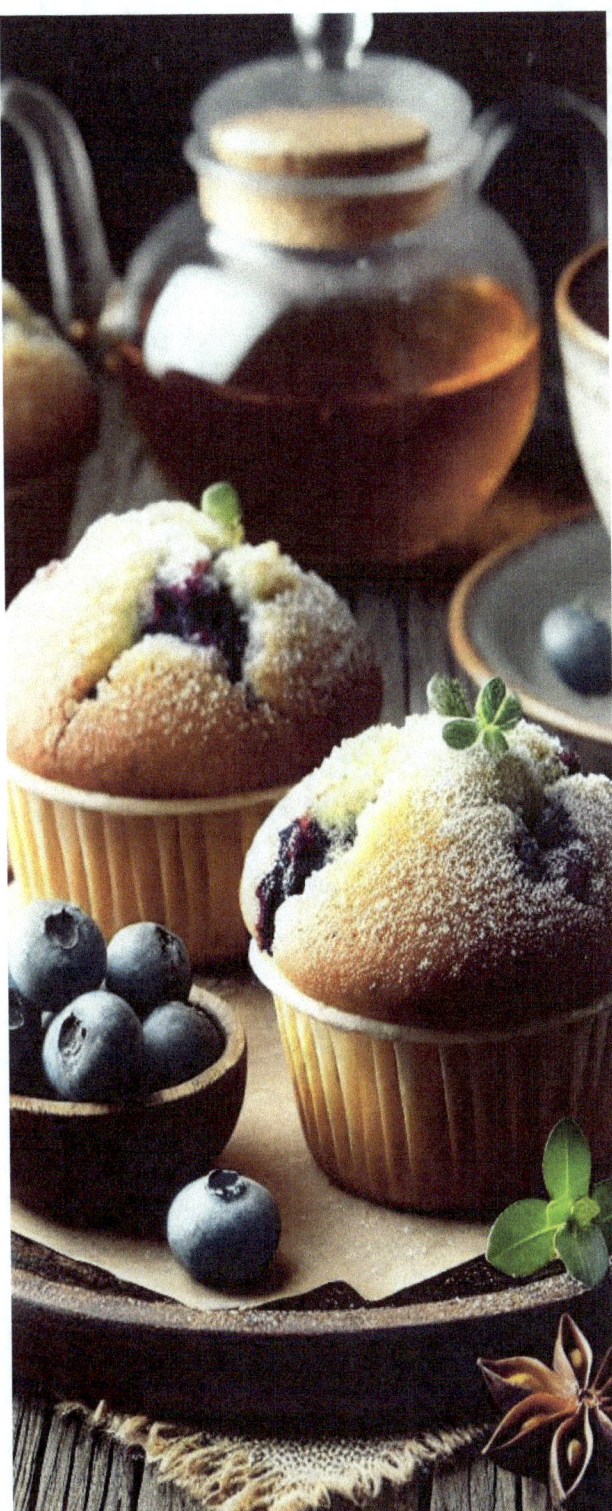

- 1 1/2 cups almond flour
- 1/4 cup coconut flour
- 1/4 teaspoon baking soda
- 1/2 teaspoon cinnamon
- 2 large eggs
- 1/4 cup unsweetened almond milk
- 1/4 cup honey
- 1 teaspoon vanilla extract
- 1/2 cup fresh blueberries

Instructions:

- Preheat the oven to 350°F (175°C). Line a muffin tin with paper liners or lightly grease.
- In a bowl, whisk together the almond flour, coconut flour, baking soda, and cinnamon.
- In another bowl, whisk the eggs, almond milk, honey, and vanilla extract until smooth.
- Stir the wet ingredients into the dry ingredients until fully combined.
- Gently fold in the blueberries.
- Divide the batter evenly between the muffin cups.
- Bake for 20-25 minutes, or until a toothpick inserted into the center comes out clean.
- Let the muffins cool in the tin for 10 minutes before transferring to a wire rack to cool completely.

Nutritional Information (per serving):

- Calories: 180
- Protein: 5g
- Carbs: 16g
- Fiber: 5g
- Potassium: 200mg
- Sodium: 30mg

Tip: You can use frozen blueberries, but be sure to fold them in gently to avoid breaking them.

Lemon Coconut Macaroons

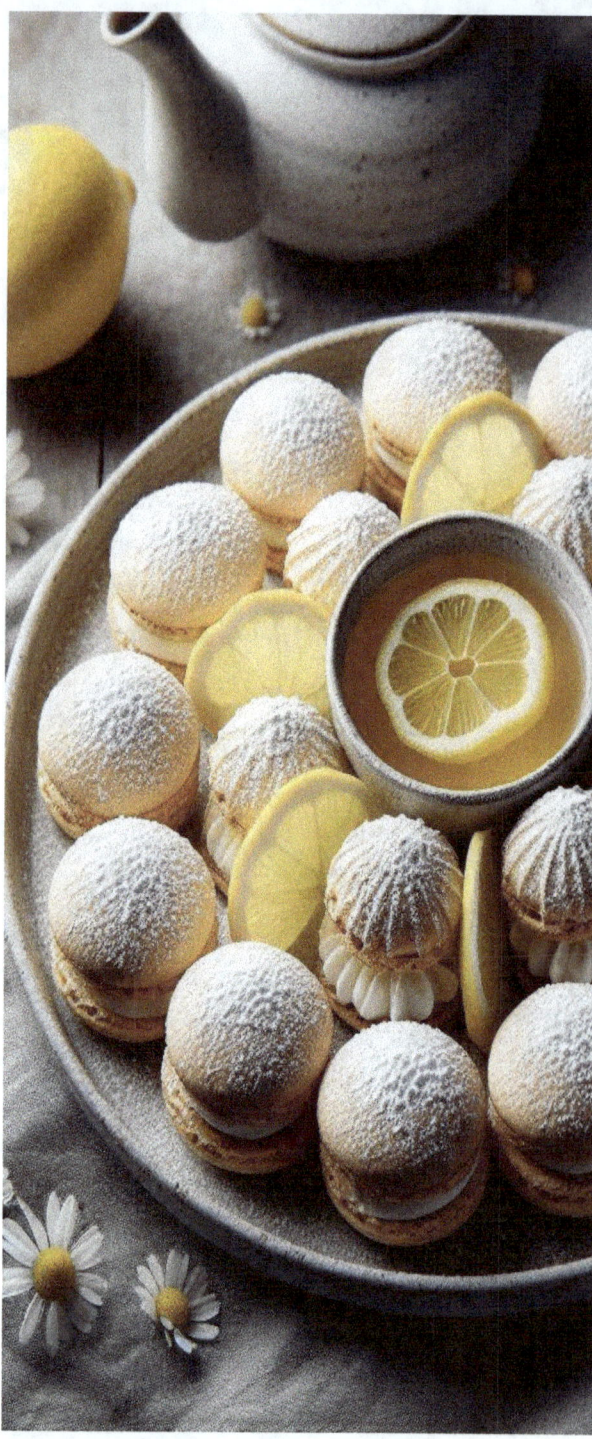

Prep Time: 15 minutes
Cooking Time: 20 minutes
Serves: 12

Ingredients:

- 2 cups unsweetened shredded coconut
- 2 large egg whites
- 1/4 cup honey or maple syrup
- 1 teaspoon lemon zest
- 1/2 teaspoon vanilla extract
- Pinch of salt

Instructions:

1. Preheat the oven to 350°F (175°C).
2. In a large bowl, whisk together the egg whites, honey, lemon zest, vanilla, and salt until frothy.
3. Add the shredded coconut to the bowl and mix until combined.
4. Scoop tablespoon-sized portions of the coconut mixture and place them on a baking sheet lined with parchment paper.
5. Bake for 18-20 minutes, until the macaroons are golden brown on the edges.
6. Let them cool on the baking sheet for 5 minutes before transferring to a wire rack to cool completely.

Nutritional Information (per serving):

- Calories: 120
- Protein: 2g
- Carbs: 15g
- Fiber: 2g
- Potassium: 90mg
- Sodium: 10mg

Tip: For a variation, dip the bottom of each macaroon in dark chocolate and let set before serving.

Rice Pudding with Stevia and Cinnamon

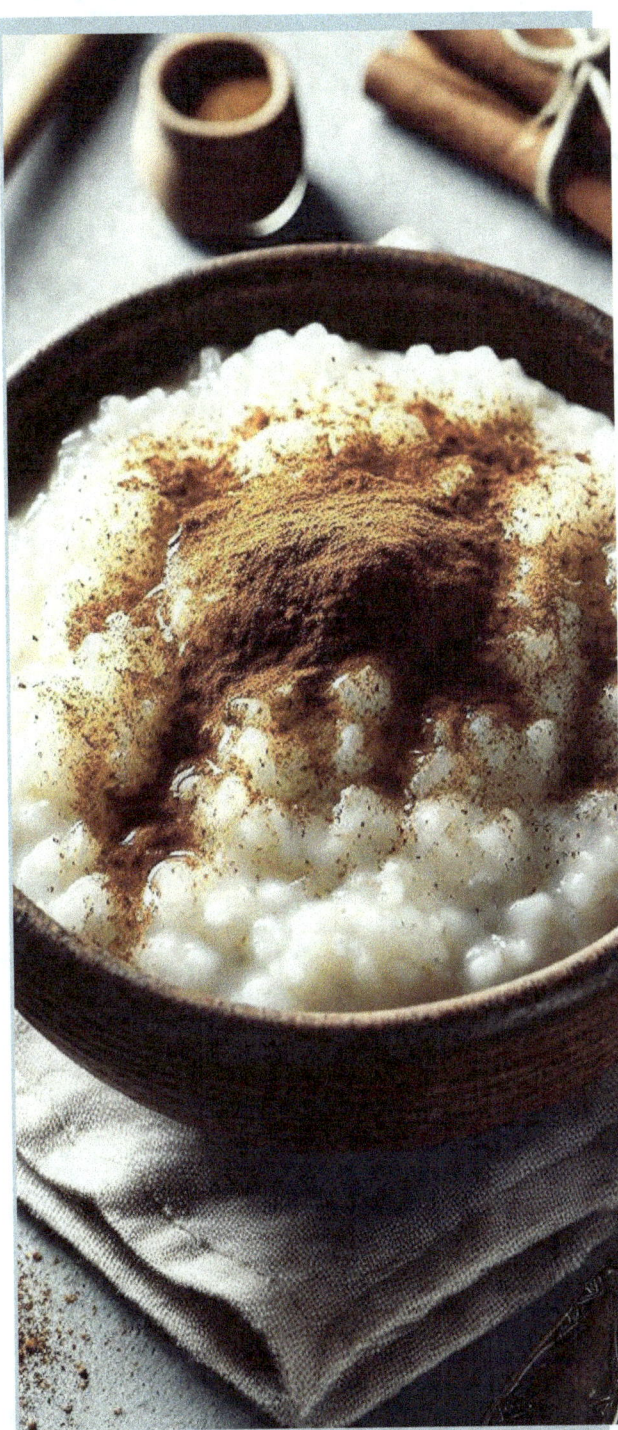

Prep Time: 10 minutes
Cooking Time: 30 minutes
Serves: 4

Ingredients:

- 1/2 cup white rice
- 2 cups unsweetened almond milk
- 1/4 teaspoon cinnamon
- 1/4 teaspoon vanilla extract
- 1 tablespoon stevia (or to taste)
- Pinch of salt

Instructions:

1. In a medium saucepan, combine the rice, almond milk, cinnamon, vanilla extract, stevia, and salt.
2. Bring to a simmer over medium heat, then reduce to low.
3. Cook for 20-30 minutes, stirring occasionally, until the rice is tender and the mixture has thickened to a pudding-like consistency.
4. Remove from heat and let cool for a few minutes before serving.
5. Sprinkle with additional cinnamon before serving, if desired.

Nutritional Information (per serving):

- Calories: 150
- Protein: 3g
- Carbs: 28g
- Fiber: 2g
- Potassium: 180mg
- Sodium: 40mg

Tip: For a creamier texture, add a bit more almond milk while cooking, or use full-fat coconut milk instead of almond milk.

Frozen Banana Bites with Dark Chocolate

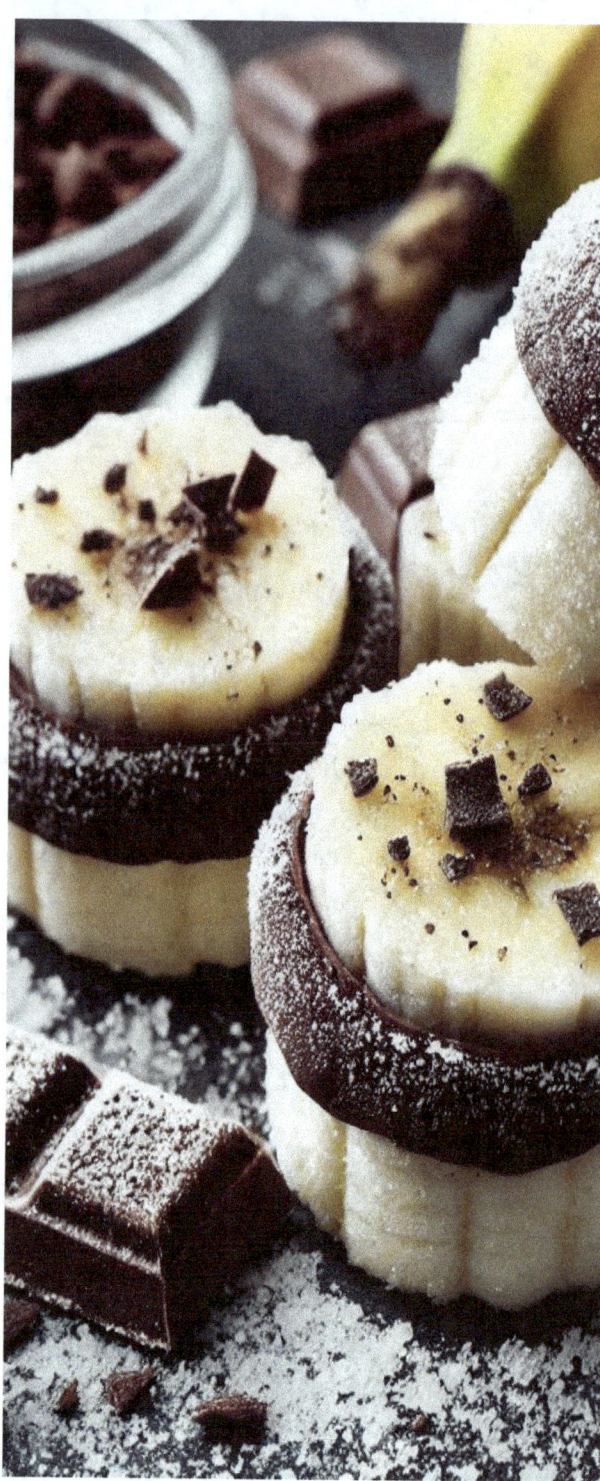

Prep Time: 10 minutes
Cooking Time: 0 minutes
Serves: 6

Ingredients:

- 2 ripe bananas, sliced
- 1/2 cup dark chocolate (at least 70% cocoa), melted
- 1/4 cup unsweetened shredded coconut (optional)

Instructions:

1. Lay the banana slices on a baking sheet lined with parchment paper.
2. Dip each slice into the melted dark chocolate, ensuring it is fully coated.
3. Sprinkle with shredded coconut, if desired.
4. Freeze the banana bites for 1-2 hours, or until the chocolate is firm.
5. Serve cold, and enjoy a sweet, refreshing treat.

Nutritional Information (per serving):

- Calories: 140
- Protein: 2g
- Carbs: 30g
- Fiber: 4g
- Potassium: 400mg
- Sodium: 5mg

Tip: Use a toothpick to dip the banana slices into the chocolate for less mess.

Baked Apples with Almond Stuffing

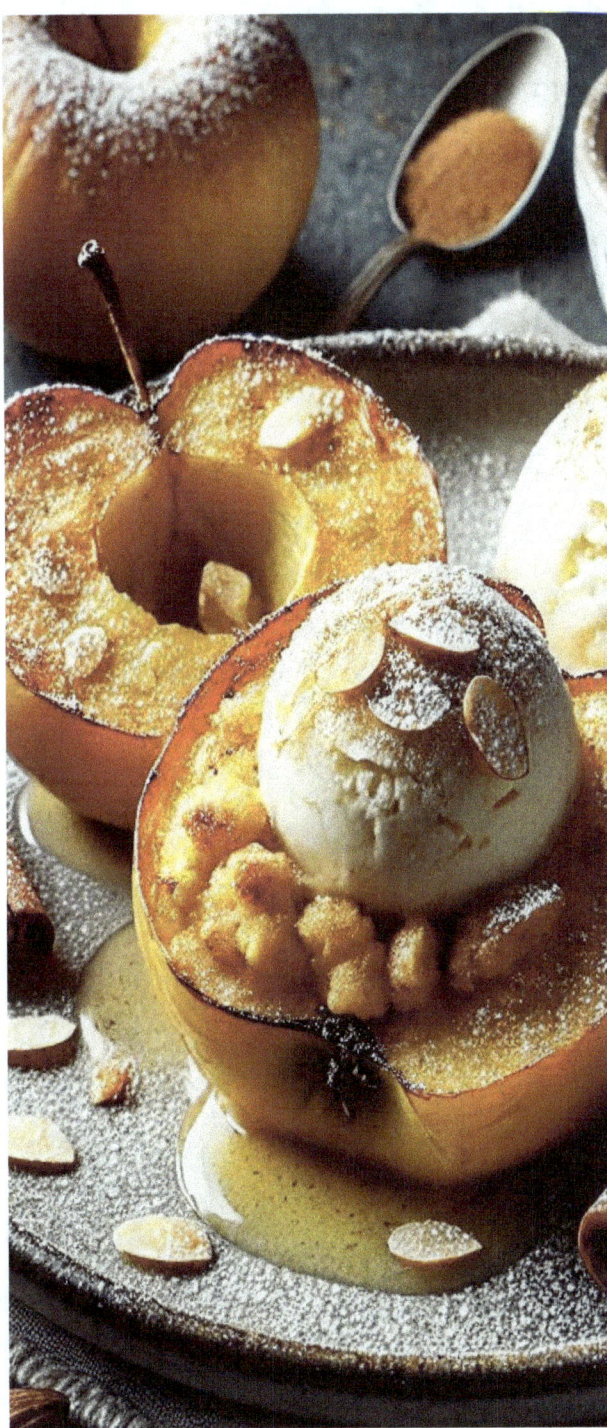

Prep Time: 15 minutes
Cooking Time: 35 minutes
Serves: 4

Ingredients:

- 4 medium apples, cored
- 1/4 cup almond flour
- 1/4 cup chopped almonds
- 2 tablespoons honey
- 1/2 teaspoon cinnamon
- 1/4 teaspoon nutmeg

Instructions:

1. Preheat the oven to 350°F (175°C).
2. In a small bowl, mix the almond flour, chopped almonds, honey, cinnamon, and nutmeg to make the stuffing.
3. Stuff each apple with the almond mixture and place them in a baking dish.
4. Bake for 30-35 minutes, until the apples are tender.
5. Serve warm, optionally with a dollop of unsweetened whipped cream or yogurt.

Nutritional Information (per serving):

- Calories: 170
- Protein: 4g
- Carbs: 30g
- Fiber: 6g
- Potassium: 250mg
- Sodium: 5mg

Tip: If you prefer a sweeter version, add a bit more honey or maple syrup to the stuffing.

Raspberry Sorbet with a Lemon Twist

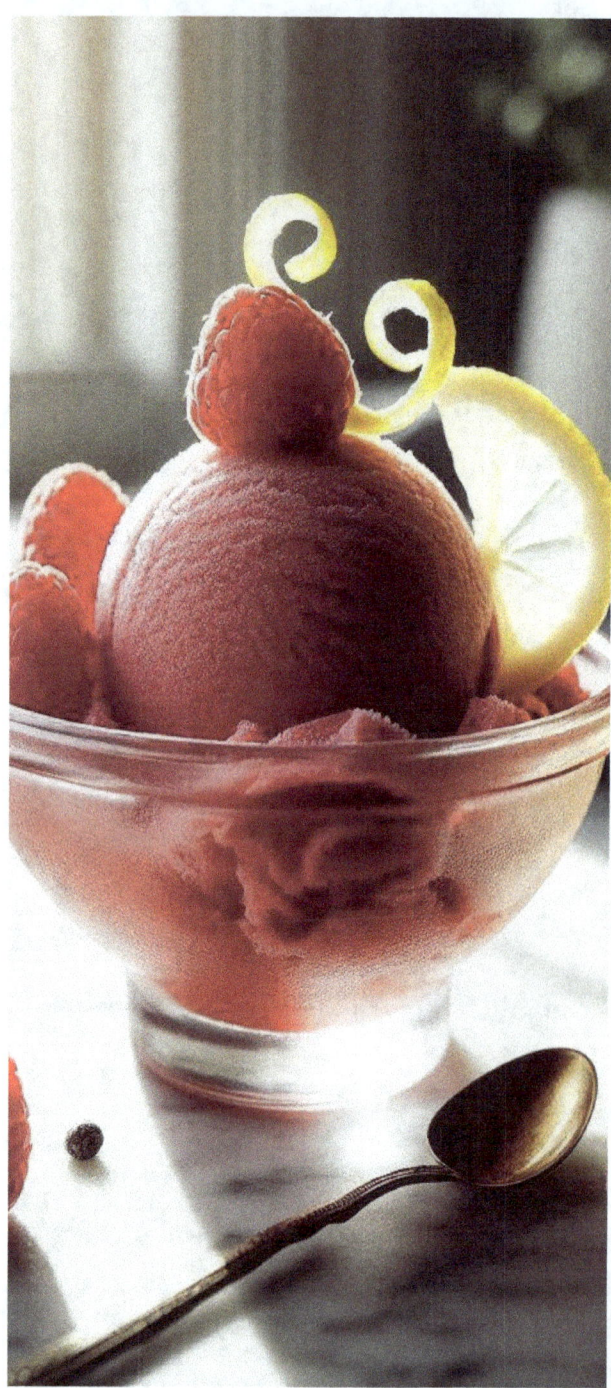

Prep Time: 5 minutes
Cooking Time: 0 minutes
Serves: 4

Ingredients:

- 2 cups fresh raspberries
- 1/4 cup lemon juice
- 2 tablespoons honey or maple syrup
- 1/4 cup water

Instructions:

1. Combine raspberries, lemon juice, honey, and water in a blender.
2. Blend until smooth, then pour the mixture into a shallow dish.
3. Freeze for 2-3 hours, stirring every 30 minutes to create a fluffy texture.
4. Once frozen, scrape the sorbet with a fork to serve.

Nutritional Information (per serving):

- Calories: 90
- Protein: 1g
- Carbs: 22g
- Fiber: 5g
- Potassium: 160mg
- Sodium: 5mg

Tip: Add a few fresh mint leaves for garnish and a burst of refreshing flavor.

Homemade Apple Pie with a Nut Crust

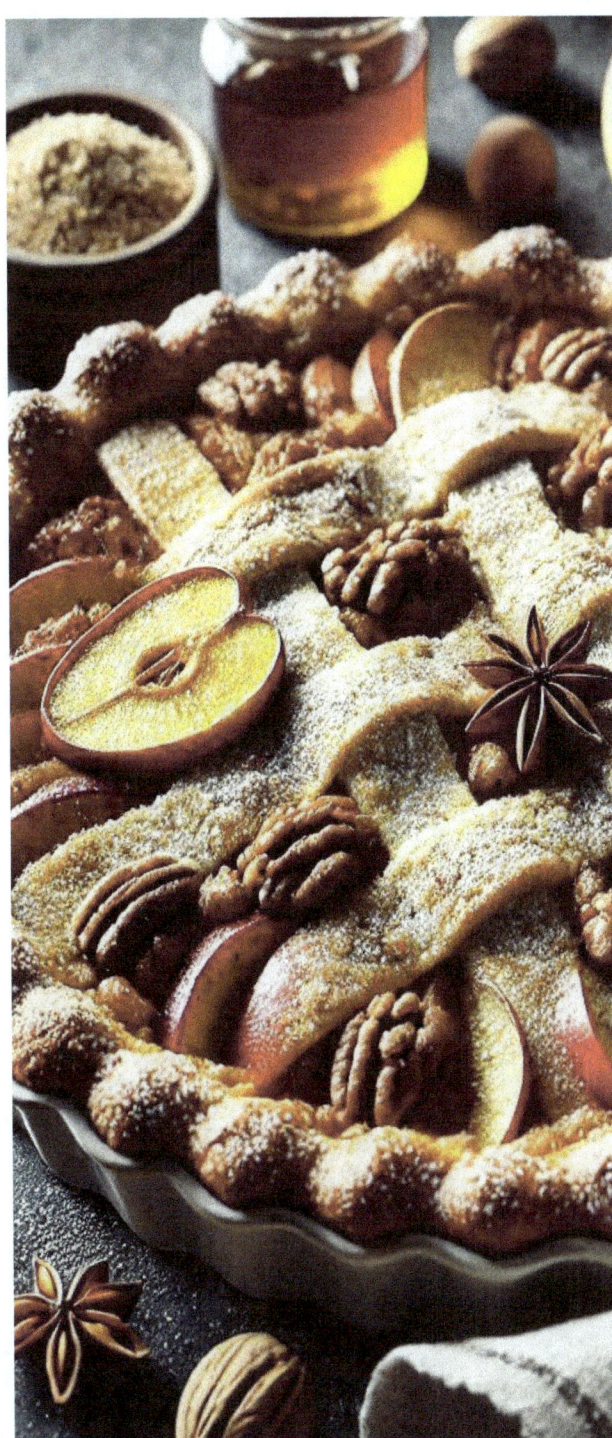

Prep Time: 20 minutes

Cooking Time: 45 minutes

Serves: 8

Ingredients:

- 4 medium apples, peeled and sliced
- 1 tablespoon lemon juice
- 1/4 cup honey or maple syrup
- 1/4 teaspoon cinnamon
- 1/4 teaspoon nutmeg
- 1/2 cup almond flour
- 1/4 cup chopped pecans
- 2 tablespoons coconut oil, melted

Instructions:

1. Preheat the oven to 350°F (175°C).
2. Toss the apple slices with lemon juice, honey, cinnamon, and nutmeg, then place them in a pie dish.
3. In a small bowl, combine almond flour, chopped pecans, and melted coconut oil to make the crust.
4. Sprinkle the crust mixture over the apples.
5. Bake for 40-45 minutes, until the apples are tender and the crust is golden brown.
6. Let cool before serving.

Nutritional Information (per serving):

- Calories: 160
- Protein: 4g
- Carbs: 22g
- Fiber: 5g
- Potassium: 180mg
- Sodium: 5mg

Tip: Serve with a scoop of low-sodium vanilla ice cream for an extra indulgence.

Chapter 7

Snacks

Carrot Sticks with Low-Sodium Hummus

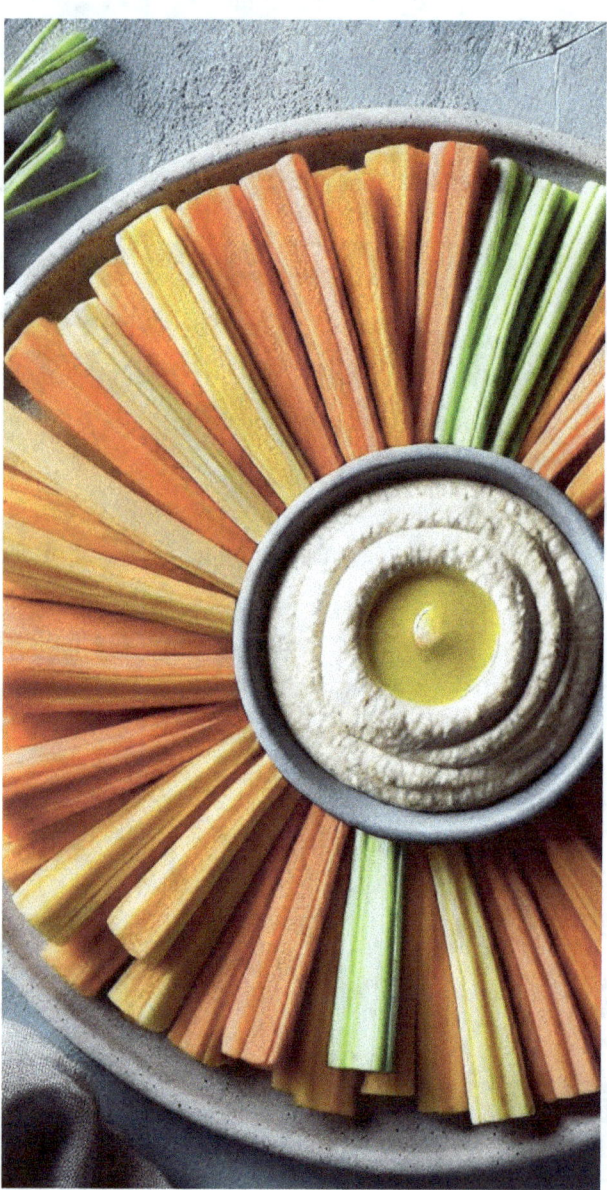

Prep Time: 5 minutes
Cooking Time: 0 minutes
Serves: 2
Ingredients:

- 2 large carrots, peeled and cut into sticks
- 1/2 cup low-sodium hummus

Instructions:

- Peel the carrots and cut them into thin sticks.
- Serve the carrot sticks with a small bowl of low-sodium hummus for dipping.

Nutritional Information (per serving):

- Calories: 90
- Protein: 3g
- Carbs: 18g
- Fiber: 5g
- Potassium: 350mg
- Sodium: 50mg

Tip: For an extra crunch, try adding a sprinkle of cumin or paprika to your hummus.

Baked Kale Chips with Olive Oil and Lemon

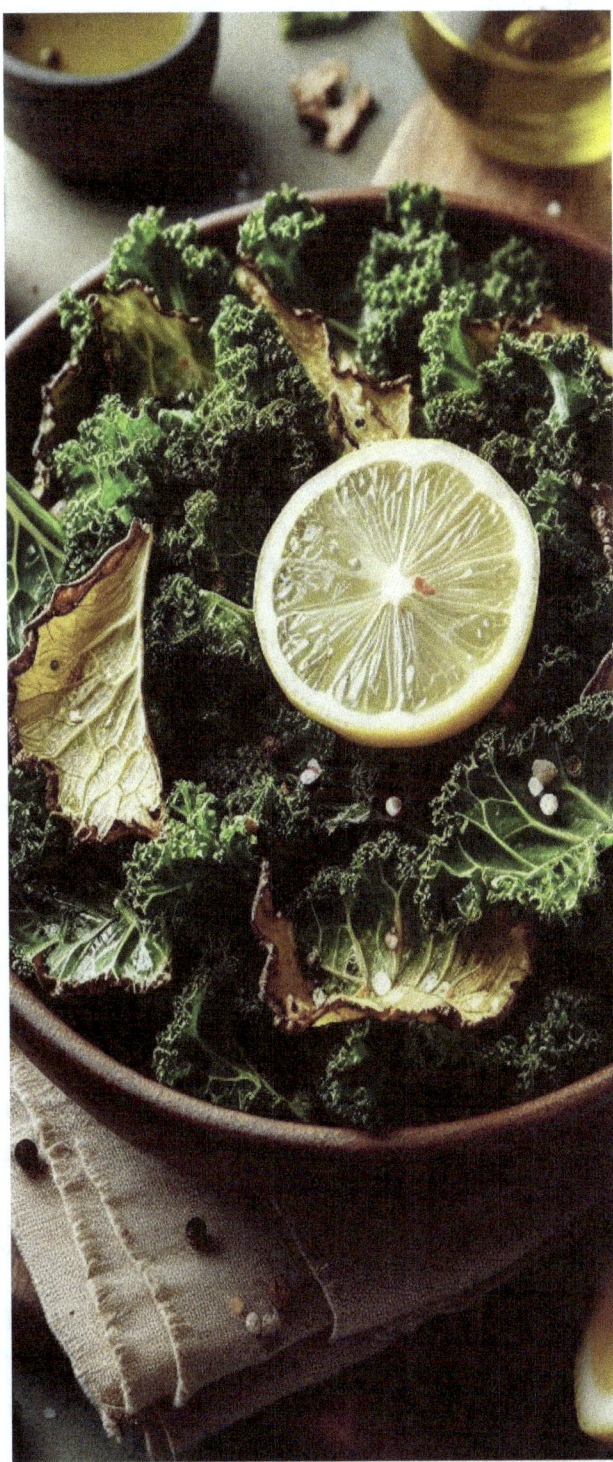

Prep Time: 10 minutes
Cooking Time: 15 minutes
Serves: 4
Ingredients:

- 1 bunch kale, washed and dried
- 1 tablespoon olive oil
- 1/2 teaspoon sea salt
- 1 teaspoon lemon juice

Instructions:

- Preheat the oven to 350°F (175°C).
- Tear the kale leaves into bite-sized pieces, discarding the tough stems.
- Toss the kale with olive oil, sea salt, and lemon juice.
- Spread the kale evenly on a baking sheet.
- Bake for 10-15 minutes, or until the kale is crispy but not burnt.
- Serve immediately.

Nutritional Information (per serving):

- Calories: 50
- Protein: 1g
- Carbs: 8g
- Fiber: 3g
- Potassium: 300mg
- Sodium: 150mg

Tip: For a spicy kick, sprinkle with a pinch of chili flakes before baking.

Rice Cakes with Almond Butter and Cucumber

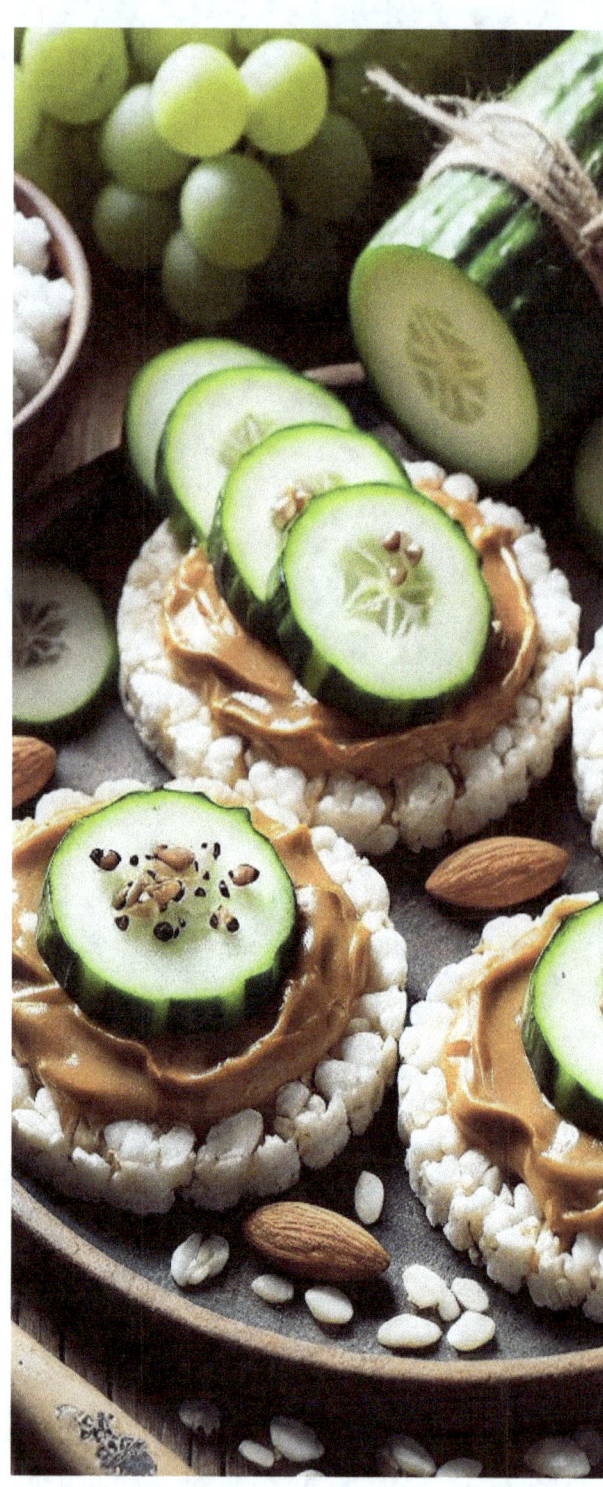

Prep Time: 5 minutes
Cooking Time: 0 minutes
Serves: 2
Ingredients:

- 2 plain rice cakes
- 2 tablespoons almond butter
- 1/2 cucumber, thinly sliced

Instructions:

- Spread almond butter evenly over each rice cake.
- Arrange cucumber slices on top of the almond butter.
- Serve immediately as a quick snack.

Nutritional Information (per serving):

- Calories: 150
- Protein: 5g
- Carbs: 18g
- Fiber: 4g
- Potassium: 180mg
- Sodium: 0mg

Tip: For extra flavor, sprinkle with a dash of ground cinnamon or a few sesame seeds.

Cucumber and Tomato Salad with Olive Oil

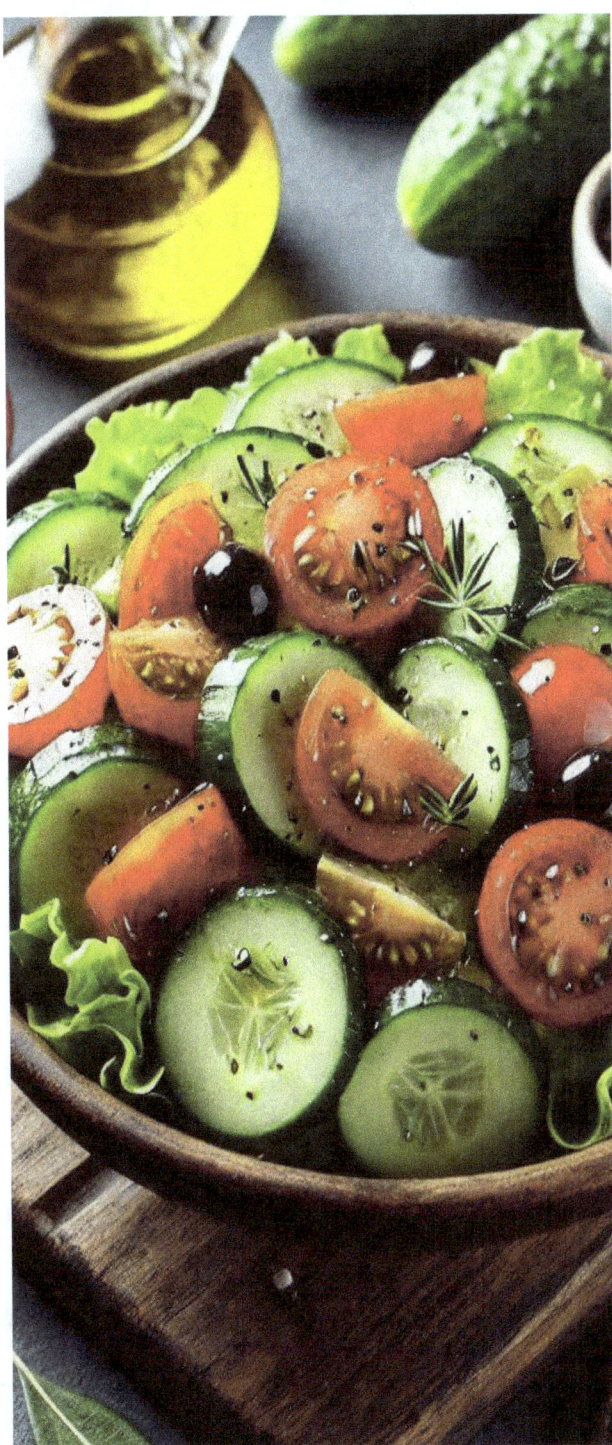

Prep Time: 5 minutes

Cooking Time: 0 minutes

Serves: 2

Ingredients:

- 1 cucumber, sliced
- 1 tomato, diced
- 1 tablespoon olive oil
- 1 teaspoon lemon juice
- Fresh parsley, chopped
- Salt and pepper, to taste

Instructions:

- Combine the cucumber and tomato in a bowl.
- Drizzle with olive oil and lemon juice.
- Season with salt and pepper, then toss to combine.
- Garnish with fresh parsley and serve.

Nutritional Information (per serving):

- Calories: 80
- Protein: 2g
- Carbs: 6g
- Fiber: 2g
- Potassium: 330mg
- Sodium: 60mg

Tip: Add a sprinkle of feta or goat cheese for a creamy texture if desired.

Greek Yogurt with Berries and Chia Seeds

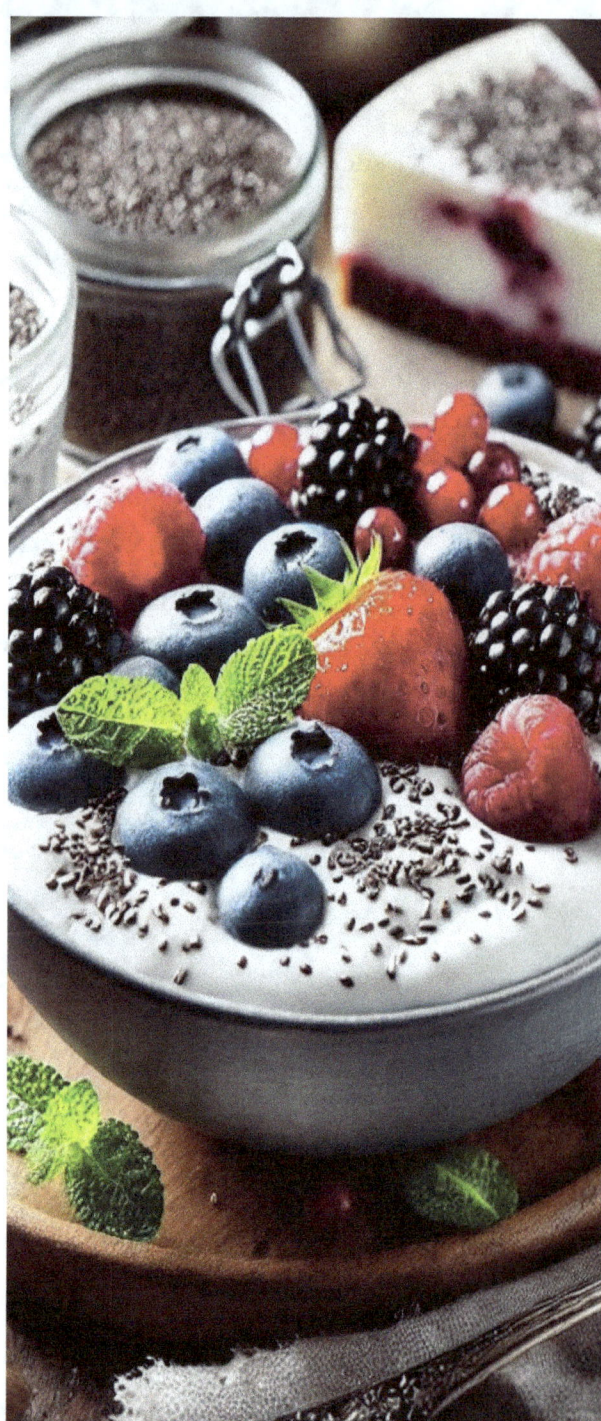

Prep Time: 5 minutes
Cooking Time: 0 minutes
Serves: 2
Ingredients:

- 1 cup plain Greek yogurt (low-fat or non-fat)
- 1/2 cup mixed berries (blueberries, strawberries, raspberries)
- 1 tablespoon chia seeds

Instructions:

- Spoon the Greek yogurt into a bowl.
- Top with mixed berries and sprinkle chia seeds on top.
- Serve immediately.

Nutritional Information (per serving):

- Calories: 120
- Protein: 10g
- Carbs: 12g
- Fiber: 5g
- Potassium: 300mg
- Sodium: 40mg

Tip: If you prefer a sweeter snack, drizzle with a small amount of honey or maple syrup.

Homemade Veggie Chips with Sweet Potato and Zucchini

Prep Time: 10 minutes
Cooking Time: 20 minutes
Serves: 4
Ingredients:

- 1 medium sweet potato, thinly sliced
- 1 medium zucchini, thinly sliced
- 1 tablespoon olive oil
- 1/2 teaspoon paprika
- Salt, to taste

Instructions:

- Preheat the oven to 375°F (190°C).
- Toss the sweet potato and zucchini slices with olive oil, paprika, and salt.
- Arrange the slices in a single layer on a baking sheet.
- Bake for 15-20 minutes, flipping halfway through, until crispy.
- Let cool slightly before serving.

Nutritional Information (per serving):

- Calories: 90
- Protein: 2g
- Carbs: 20g
- Fiber: 4g
- Potassium: 600mg
- Sodium: 100mg

Tip: Experiment with other vegetables like carrots or parsnips for variety.

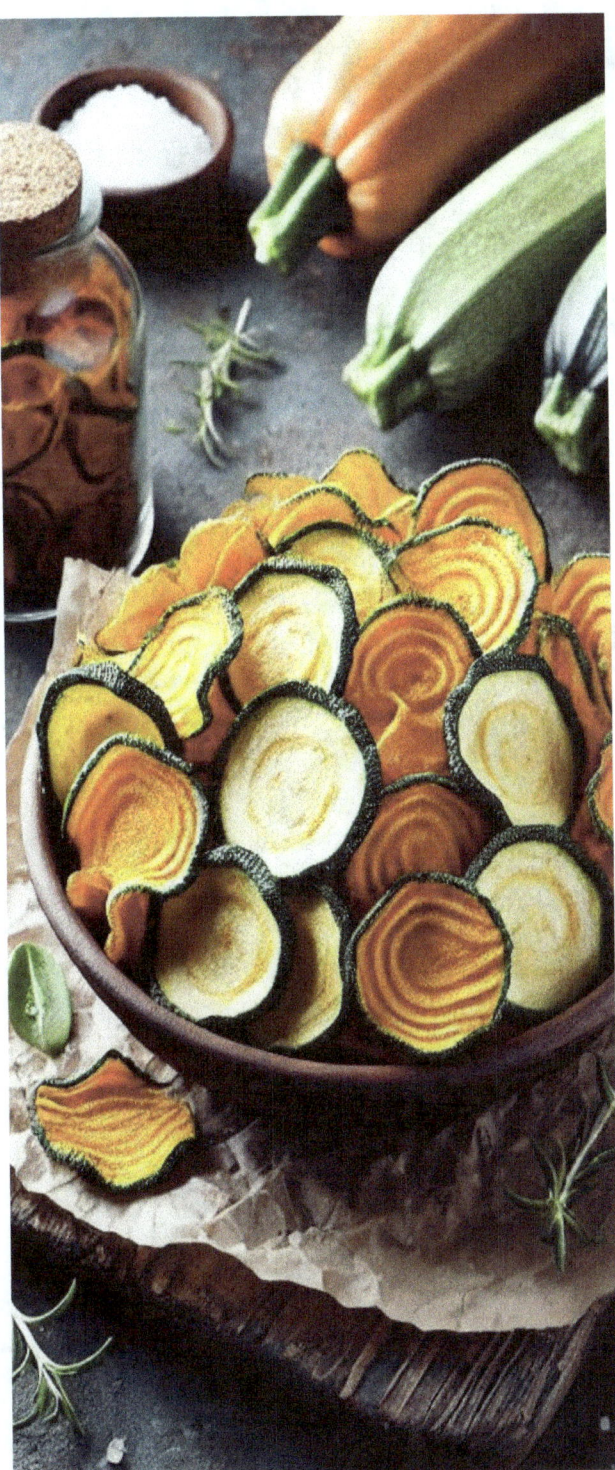

Air-Fried Sweet Potato Fries

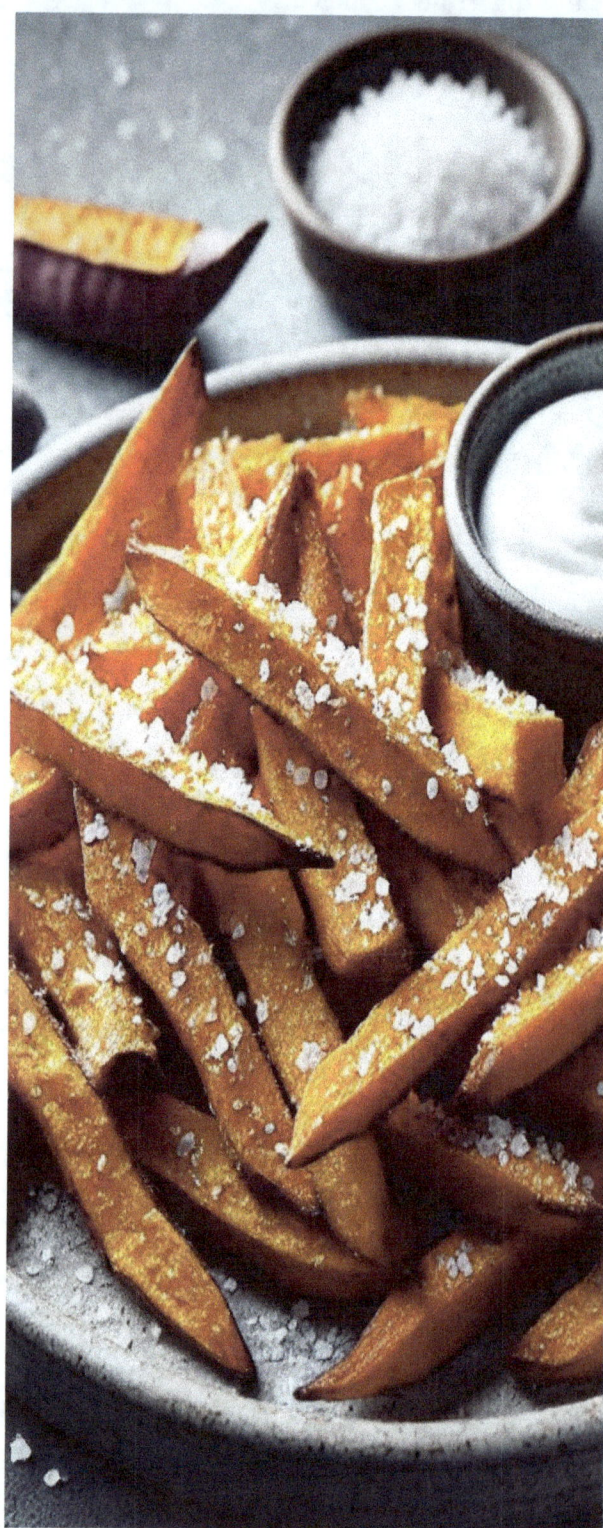

Prep Time: 5 minutes
Cooking Time: 15 minutes
Serves: 2
Ingredients:

- 2 medium sweet potatoes, cut into fries
- 1 tablespoon olive oil
- 1/2 teaspoon smoked paprika
- Salt and pepper, to taste

Instructions:

- Preheat the air fryer to 375°F (190°C).
- Toss the sweet potato fries with olive oil, smoked paprika, salt, and pepper.
- Place the fries in the air fryer basket and cook for 12-15 minutes, shaking halfway through.
- Serve hot.

Nutritional Information (per serving):

- Calories: 140
- Protein: 2g
- Carbs: 30g
- Fiber: 5g
- Potassium: 700mg
- Sodium: 120mg

Tip: Serve with a side of low-sodium ketchup or Greek yogurt for dipping.

Cottage Cheese with Pineapple

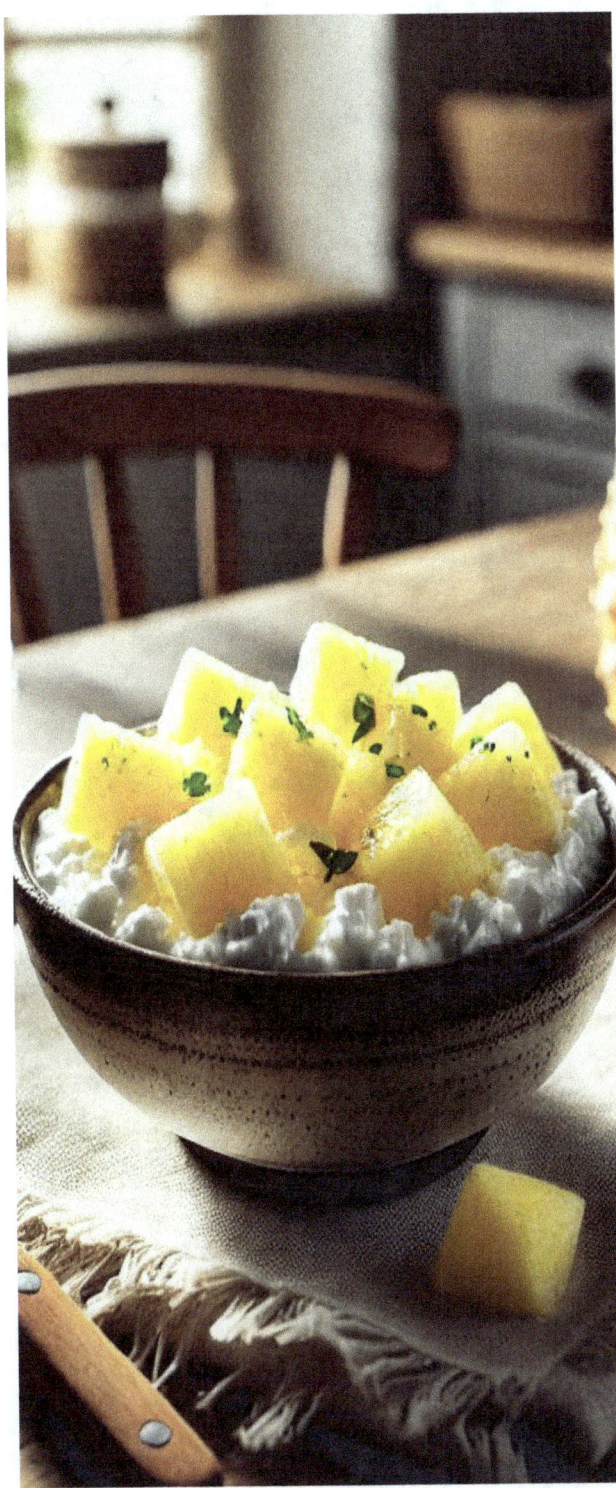

Prep Time: 5 minutes

Cooking Time: 0 minutes

Serves: 1

Ingredients:

- 1/2 cup low-fat cottage cheese
- 1/2 cup fresh pineapple chunks

Instructions:

- Spoon the cottage cheese into a bowl.
- Top with fresh pineapple chunks.
- Serve immediately.

Nutritional Information (per serving):

- Calories: 150
- Protein: 12g
- Carbs: 18g
- Fiber: 2g
- Potassium: 150mg
- Sodium: 200mg

Tip: If you prefer a sweeter snack, drizzle a little honey or stevia over the top.

Almonds and Fresh Strawberries

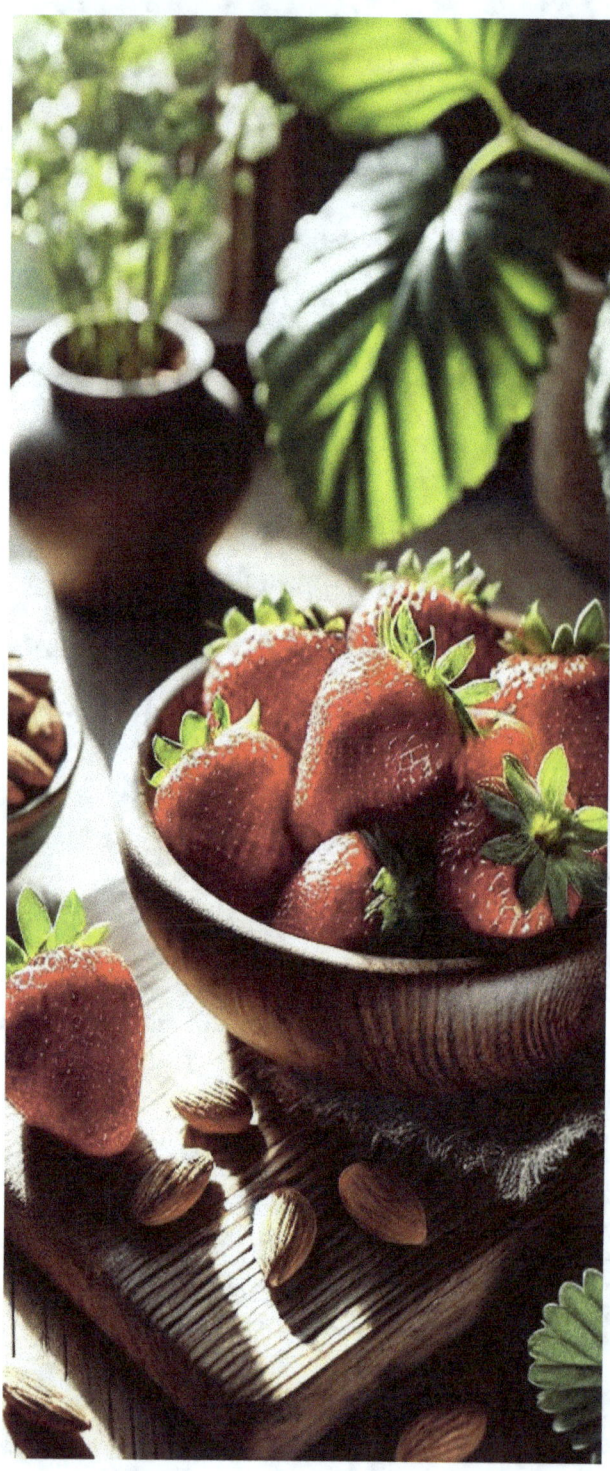

Prep Time: 5 minutes
Cooking Time: 0 minutes
Serves: 1
Ingredients:

- 1/4 cup almonds
- 1/2 cup fresh strawberries, halved

Instructions:

- Arrange the almonds and strawberries on a plate.
- Serve immediately as a light, satisfying snack.

Nutritional Information (per serving):

- Calories: 170
- Protein: 5g
- Carbs: 15g
- Fiber: 4g
- Potassium: 300mg
- Sodium: 0mg

Tip: Pair with a glass of water or herbal tea for added hydration.

Apple Slices with Almond Butter

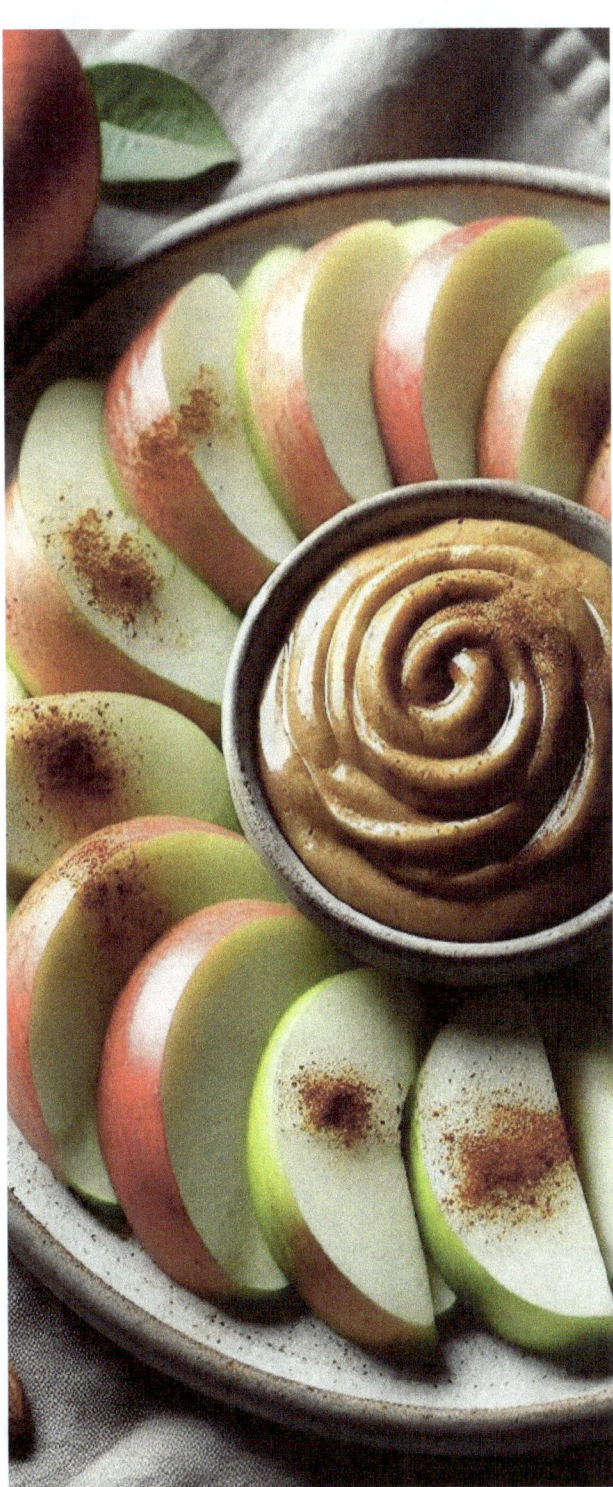

Prep Time: 5 minutes

Cooking Time: 0 minutes

Serves: 1

Ingredients:

- 1 apple, sliced
- 2 tablespoons almond butter

Instructions:

1. Slice the apple into thin wedges.
2. Dip the apple slices into almond butter and enjoy.

Nutritional Information (per serving):

- Calories: 200
- Protein: 5g
- Carbs: 28g
- Fiber: 5g
- Potassium: 240mg
- Sodium: 0mg

Tip: Add a sprinkle of cinnamon or nutmeg for extra flavor.

Roasted Chickpeas with Paprika

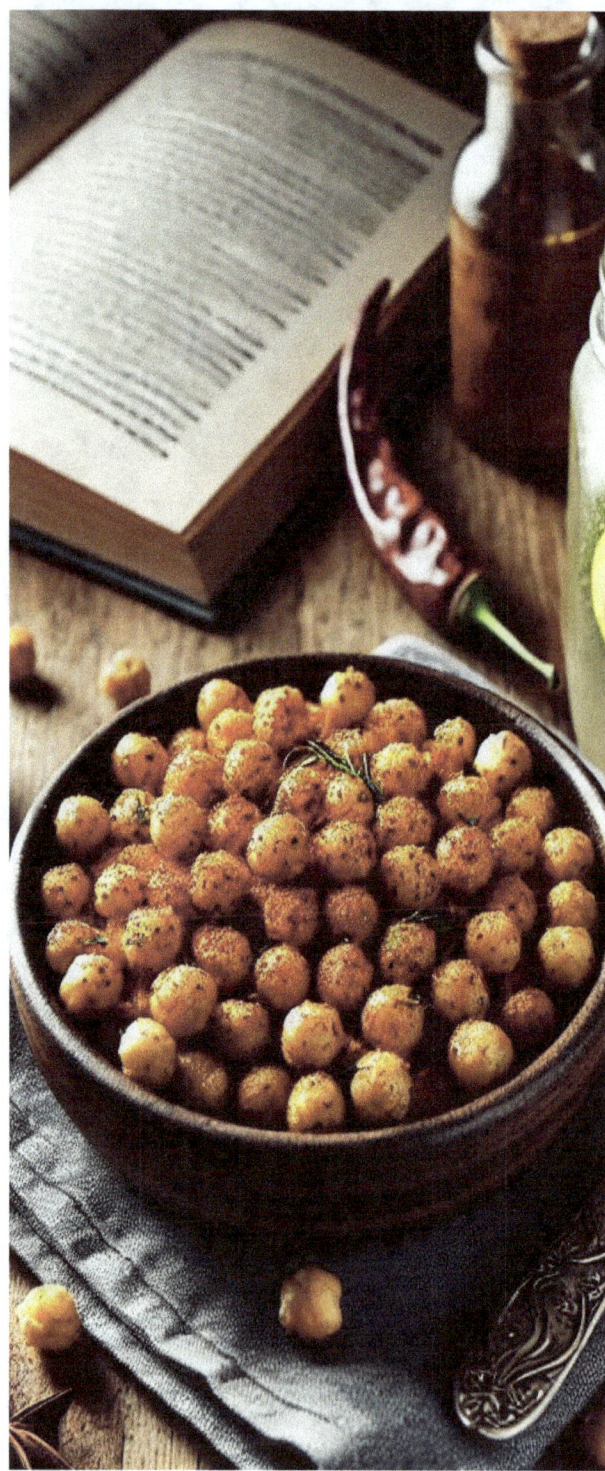

Prep Time: 10 minutes

Cooking Time: 30 minutes

Serves: 4

Ingredients:

- 1 can (15 oz) chickpeas, drained and rinsed
- 1 tablespoon olive oil
- 1/2 teaspoon paprika
- Salt to taste

Instructions:

1. Preheat the oven to 400°F (200°C).
2. Toss chickpeas with olive oil, paprika, and salt.
3. Spread them in a single layer on a baking sheet.
4. Roast for 25-30 minutes, shaking the pan halfway through.
5. Serve as a crunchy, savory snack.

Nutritional Information (per serving):

- Calories: 120
- Protein: 6g
- Carbs: 20g
- Fiber: 5g
- Potassium: 350mg
- Sodium: 150mg

Tip: Experiment with other seasonings like garlic powder or cumin.

Peach and Mint Salad

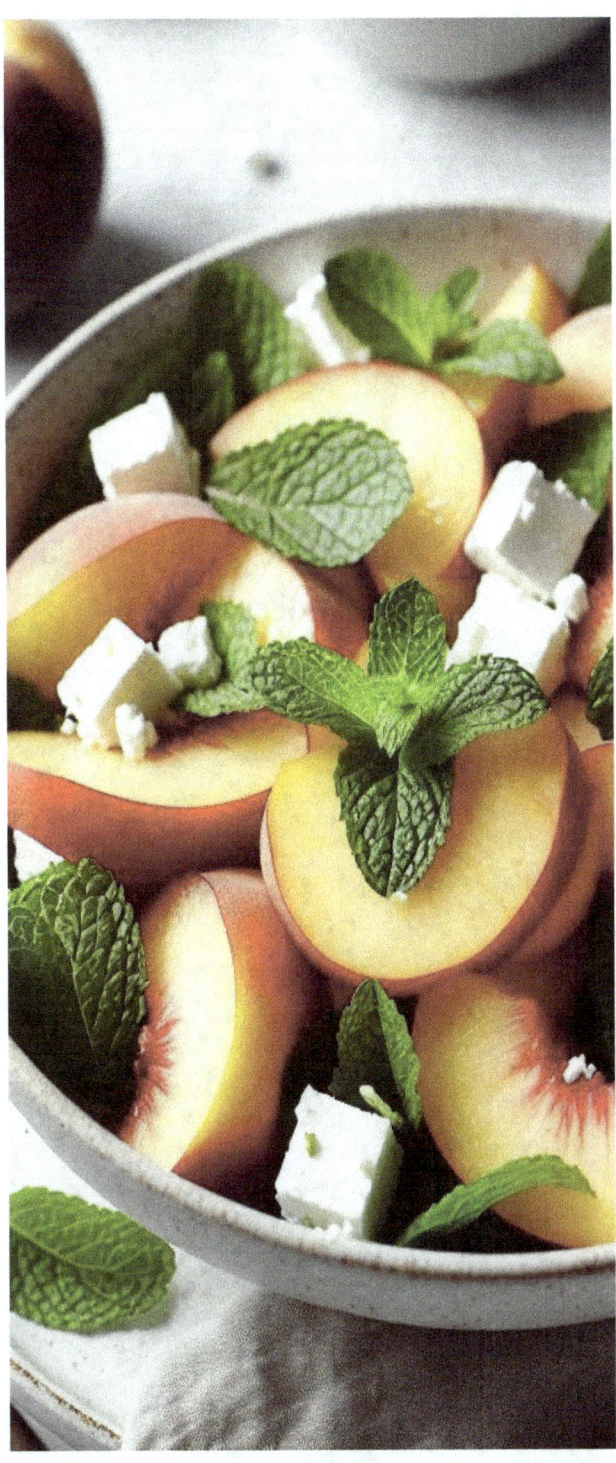

Prep Time: 10 minutes

Cooking Time: 0 minutes

Serves: 2

Ingredients:

- 2 fresh peaches, sliced
- 1/4 cup fresh mint leaves, chopped
- 1 tablespoon honey (optional)

Instructions:

1. Slice the peaches and arrange them on a plate.
2. Sprinkle the chopped mint leaves over the top.
3. Drizzle with honey if desired, and serve immediately.

Nutritional Information (per serving):

- Calories: 80
- Protein: 1g
- Carbs: 20g
- Fiber: 3g
- Potassium: 250mg
- Sodium: 0mg

Tip: Serve chilled for a refreshing summer snack.

Low-Sodium Tuna with Cucumber Slices

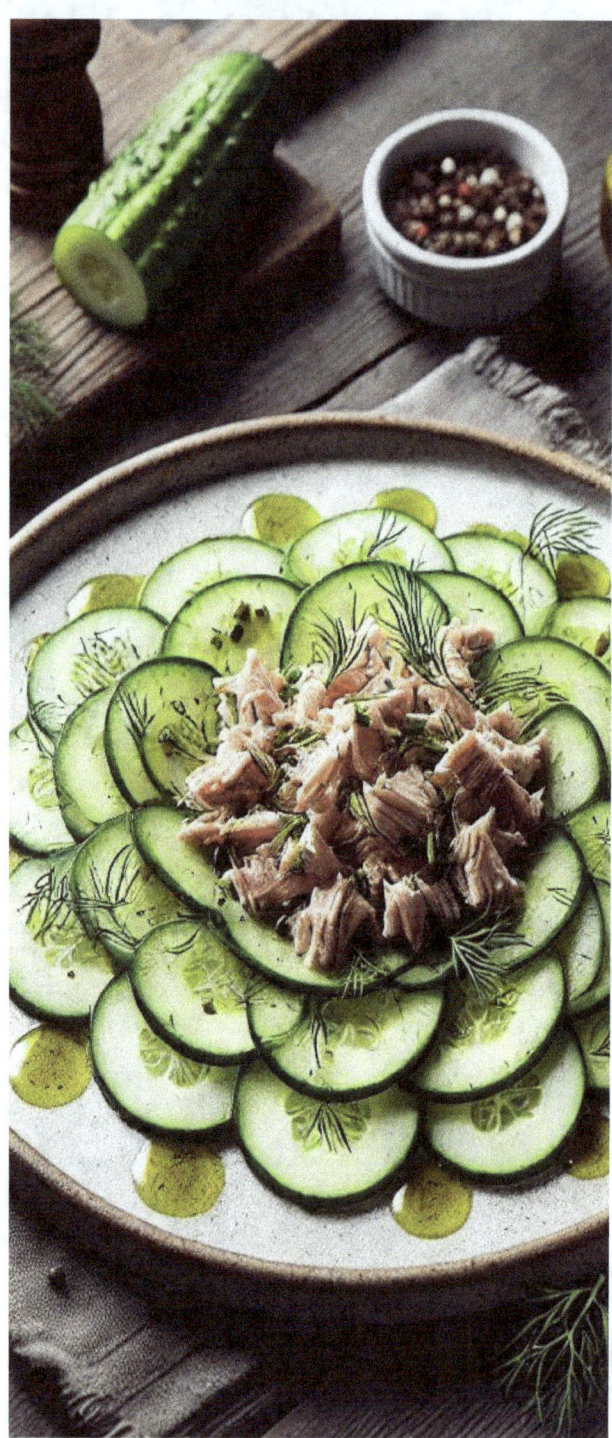

Prep Time: 5 minutes

Cooking Time: 0 minutes

Serves: 1

Ingredients:

- 1 can (5 oz) low-sodium tuna, drained
- 1/2 cucumber, sliced

Instructions:

1. Mix the drained tuna with a dash of olive oil or lemon juice.
2. Serve with fresh cucumber slices for a quick, savory bite.

Nutritional Information (per serving):

- Calories: 140
- Protein: 20g
- Carbs: 2g
- Fiber: 1g
- Potassium: 250mg
- Sodium: 100mg

Tip: Add a sprinkle of pepper or a squeeze of lemon for extra zest.

Rice and Apple Salad with Cinnamon

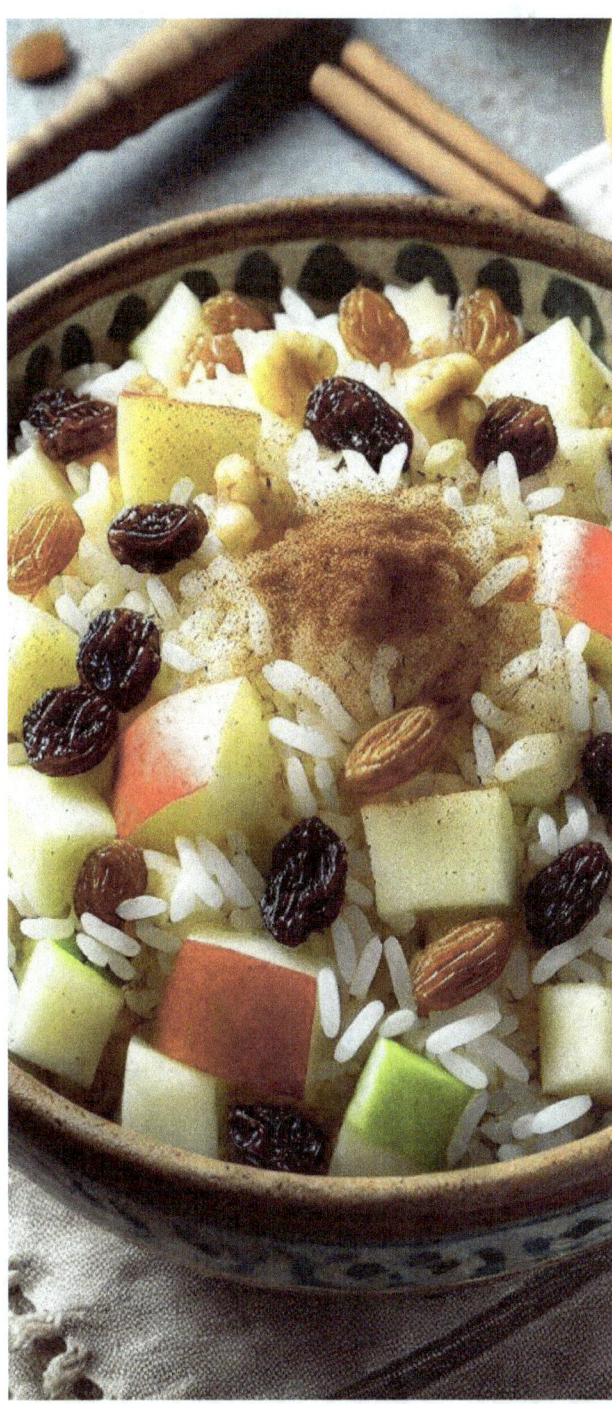

Prep Time: 10 minutes

Cooking Time: 0 minutes

Serves: 2

Ingredients:

- 1/2 cup cooked brown rice, cooled
- 1 apple, diced
- 1/4 teaspoon cinnamon
- 1 tablespoon lemon juice

Instructions:

1. In a bowl, mix the cooked rice, diced apple, cinnamon, and lemon juice.
2. Toss to combine, then serve immediately.

Nutritional Information (per serving):

- Calories: 140
- Protein: 3g
- Carbs: 30g
- Fiber: 4g
- Potassium: 200mg
- Sodium: 5mg

Tip: Add a few chopped nuts for added crunch and flavor.

Hard-Boiled Eggs with Fresh Herbs

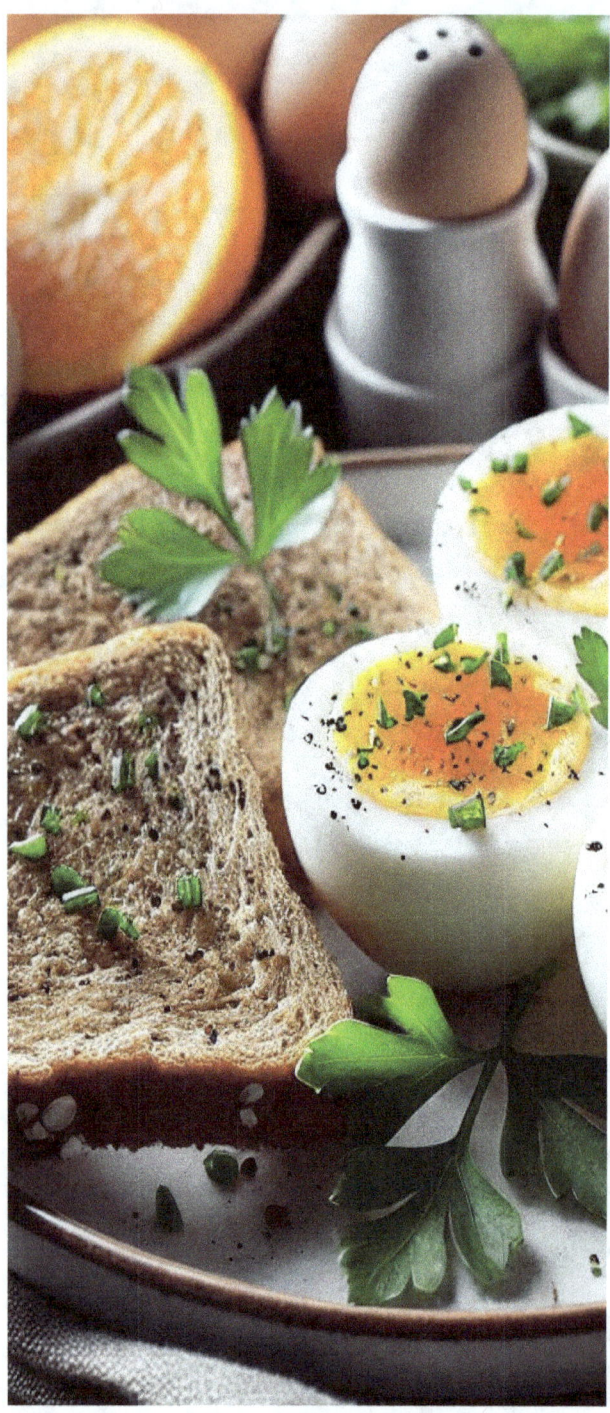

Prep Time: 5 minutes

Cooking Time: 10 minutes

Serves: 2

Ingredients:

- 4 eggs
- Fresh herbs (parsley, chives, or dill), chopped
- Salt and pepper to taste

Instructions:

1. Boil the eggs in water for 10 minutes, then cool and peel them.
2. Slice the eggs and sprinkle with fresh herbs, salt, and pepper.
3. Serve as a protein-packed snack.

Nutritional Information (per serving):

- Calories: 140
- Protein: 12g
- Carbs: 1g
- Fiber: 0g
- Potassium: 150mg
- Sodium: 60mg

Tip: For a different twist, try adding a dash of smoked paprika or a few drops of hot sauce.

Chapter 8
Meal Prep & Time-Saving Tips

In our everyday life, treating renal illness might seem daunting. The dietary adjustments that are necessary to maintain one's health may seem to be overwhelming, and the amount of time that is needed to prepare meals that are kidney-friendly may add additional stress. On the other hand, if you use the appropriate methods, meal preparation may become a very useful tool for reducing the stress associated with daily cooking and ensuring that you adhere to your kidney-friendly diet. The trick is to make a plan ahead of time, get comfortable with cooking in batches, and make optimal use of your kitchen utensils in order to save time and effort. When you prepare meals in advance, you not only guarantee that you have the appropriate food on hand, but you also decrease the temptation to grab something fast and unhealthy when hunger hits.

The first step in meal planning for kidney health is recognizing the necessity of consistency. When you have just been diagnosed with kidney disease, it is understandable that you may be tempted to make little mistakes, particularly when you are hungry or when you are pushed for time. It will be easier for you to avoid those common errors if you have meals prepared and ready to go. In order to make eating food that is kidney-friendly simple and stress-free, let's take a look at some practical techniques to organizing your kitchen and meal planning.

Food preparation for renal illness begins with the fundamentals: planning. This is the cornerstone of effective meal preparation. Without a clear strategy in place, meal planning might seem daunting. Begin by conceiving about your meals as a sequence of simple components, each of which may be prepared in advance. The first step is to determine which meals take more time and attention, such as morning or supper, and which meals may be prepared in bulk, such as snacks or lunch. One example of the former is breakfast. Preparing meals that can be readily reheated or served cold is a time-saver. For instance, roasted vegetables, grains such as quinoa or rice, and protein-rich foods such as grilled chicken or fish may be prepared in large quantities and then portioned out for meals throughout the week.

Start your prep on a day when you have some spare time, like a Sunday afternoon, and make enough food to cover several days. A few important ingredients—like low-sodium grilled chicken, roasted sweet potatoes, or a huge quantity of quinoa—can go a long way. When you're batch cooking, think in terms of adaptable items that can be combined and matched to make multiple meals. For example, quinoa may serve as a basis for both lunch bowls and dinners, while grilled veggies can be added to salads, rice dishes, or wraps. Once these core components are available, you may toss together a variety of meals in minutes, without beginning from scratch every time.

When it comes to particular meals, breakfast may often be the toughest to get properly, especially if you're accustomed to grabbing something quick or sweet in the morning. The idea is to design meals that are simple to store and reheat. Consider creating huge amounts of low-potassium oatmeal, chia pudding, or overnight oats. These may be refrigerated in individual portions and personalized with fresh fruit, nuts, or spices when it's time to consume. Likewise, egg-based recipes, such an egg white scramble or tiny frittatas, may be cooked in advance and preserved in the refrigerator for a few days. These breakfasts not only save time but also give a nutrient-rich start to your day, setting the tone for good eating.

When bulk cooking for lunch or supper, consider about producing one-pot meals or sheet-pan recipes that need minimum labor and cleanup. For example, a chicken stir-fry with bell peppers, zucchini, and low-sodium soy sauce may be cooked in big volumes and eaten with brown rice or quinoa. You may also create a huge salad with fresh greens, topped with pre-cooked chicken or turkey and a light dressing, which will keep nicely in the fridge for a few days. If you're cooking in bulk, don't forget to divide up dishes into individual portions so they're quick to grab and go when you're ready to eat. A simple, but fulfilling dinner like baked salmon with roasted asparagus or a quinoa-stuffed bell pepper may be made ahead of time and simply kept in airtight containers for warming when required.

Time-saving equipment and kitchen gadgets may be game-changers when you're making kidney-friendly meals. A slow cooker or Instant Pot may be immensely beneficial for producing huge amounts of meals with minimum effort. These machines let you to prepare a range of meals—like soups, stews, or even chicken for salads and wraps—without having to stand over the stove. Simply set it up in the morning, and by the time you're ready for lunch or dinner, your meal will be ready and waiting. If you're not using a slow cooker, consider employing the oven for batch roasting. You can roast a variety of veggies, meats, and even grains on a single baking sheet, minimizing the amount of time you spend in the kitchen.

Another fantastic time-saving item is the food processor. It may help you chop, slice, and grate materials fast, which can be very beneficial when preparing veggies or creating things like hummus, pesto, or cauliflower rice. A mandoline slicer is another wonderful instrument for swiftly cutting veggies into uniform, thin slices, which may be beneficial for producing recipes like homemade veggie chips or zucchini noodles. If you wish to save even more time, consider investing in a meal prep container set. These containers are intended for portion management, and they enable you to keep your meals in the correct serving amounts. Having these containers ready to go helps you speed the process, and you can stack them neatly in the fridge, making your meal prep both efficient and orderly.

Another key facet of meal planning is ensuring that your supplies and meals are properly preserved. Many kidney-friendly items, including fresh vegetables and proteins, have a limited shelf life, so it's vital to store them carefully. For meats and proteins, invest in freezer-safe containers or bags to keep them fresh for longer. If you batch-cook dishes, separate them into individual servings and store them in airtight containers. Label each container with the date it was produced so you can readily monitor its freshness. For snacks like homemade vegetable chips, granola, or trail mix, put them into tiny snack-sized bags or containers for grab-and-go ease. If you're prepared fresh fruit, such as berries or melon, wash and cut them in advance, then keep them in separate containers for quick access. The more you can accomplish ahead of time, the less you'll have to worry about meal preparation throughout the week.

In addition to preserving items appropriately, consider about how to organize your pantry. Organizing your pantry with kidney-friendly basics, such as whole grains, low-sodium canned beans, dried herbs, and spices, is a terrific way to make sure you always have the correct items on hand. You don't need to spend hours food shopping—just prepare a list of the necessities and stick to it. Keeping your pantry organized will help you avoid impulse buys and ensure that you're only choosing kidney-friendly goods that correspond with your meal plan.

The most crucial component of meal preparing is making it work for your schedule and requirements. The idea is not to make meal planning a difficult or daunting activity but to incorporate it into your lifestyle in a manner that benefits your health without disturbing your day-to-day routine. By batching meals in advance, organizing your kitchen, and employing time-saving gadgets, you're setting yourself up for success. The key is consistency. By planning, cooking, and storing meals in a manner that works for you, treating kidney disease becomes not only doable but more manageable, making it simpler to maintain a kidney-friendly diet and live a happier, more balanced life.

Meal prep isn't just about cooking—it's about developing a sustainable habit that helps you keep control over your nutrition, your health, and your time. Whether you're batch cooking on weekends, utilizing your slow cooker for hands-off meals, or just arranging your fridge with easy-to-grab snacks, each step you take will make it simpler to maintain your kidney-friendly eating habits. The work you put into planning and preparing today will pay off throughout the week, helping you remain on track with your health objectives and ensuring that you have wholesome meals at your fingertips whenever you need them.

Day 1

- **Breakfast**: Low-Potassium Oatmeal with Blueberries
- **Lunch**: Grilled Chicken Salad with Olive Oil and Lemon
- **Dinner**: Baked Lemon Herb Salmon with Roasted Asparagus
- **Dessert**: Banana-Free Chocolate Avocado Mousse
- **Snack**: Carrot Sticks with Low-Sodium Hummus

Day 2

- **Breakfast**: Egg White Scramble with Spinach and Bell Peppers
- **Lunch**: Quinoa and Cucumber Salad with Greek Yogurt Dressing
- **Dinner**: Chicken Stir-Fry with Bell Peppers and Zucchini
- **Dessert**: Apple Crisp with Oats and Cinnamon
- **Snack**: Rice Cakes with Almond Butter and Cucumber

Day 3

- **Breakfast**: Chia Seed Pudding with Almond Milk and Berries
- **Lunch**: Vegetable Soup (Low-Sodium)
- **Dinner**: Grilled Turkey Burgers with Sautéed Spinach
- **Dessert**: Homemade Coconut Milk Popsicles
- **Snack**: Greek Yogurt with Berries and Chia Seeds

Day 4

- **Breakfast**: Whole Wheat Toast with Avocado and Egg
- **Lunch**: Lentil Salad with Cherry Tomatoes and Parsley
- **Dinner**: Quinoa-Stuffed Eggplant
- **Dessert**: Low-Sodium Almond Butter Cookies
- **Snack**: Homemade Veggie Chips with Sweet Potato and Zucchini

Day 5

- **Breakfast**: Apple Cinnamon Quinoa Porridge
- **Lunch**: Rice and Bean Bowl with Roasted Veggies
- **Dinner**: Baked Cod with Garlic and Roasted Brussels Sprouts
- **Dessert**: Berry Sorbet with a Touch of Lime
- **Snack**: Air-Fried Sweet Potato Fries

Day 6

- **Breakfast**: Coconut Yogurt Parfait with Low-Sodium Granola
- **Lunch**: Tuna Salad with Cabbage and Light Mayo
- **Dinner**: Low-Sodium Beef Stir Fry with Snow Peas
- **Dessert**: Chia Seed Pudding with Cacao and Almond Butter
- **Snack**: Cottage Cheese with Pineapple

Day 7

- **Breakfast**: Homemade Fruit Smoothie (Banana-Free)
- **Lunch**: Stuffed Bell Peppers with Ground Turkey and Quinoa
- **Dinner**: Chicken and Sweet Potato Mash
- **Dessert**: Carrot Cake Energy Balls
- **Snack**: Almonds and Fresh Strawberries

Day 8

- **Breakfast**: Baked Sweet Potato with Cinnamon and Walnuts
- **Lunch**: Chickpea and Spinach Stir Fry
- **Dinner**: Grilled Salmon with Steamed Broccoli and Brown Rice
- **Dessert**: Baked Pears with Cinnamon and Walnuts
- **Snack**: Apple Slices with Almond Butter

Day 9

- **Breakfast**: Zucchini Fritters with Low-Sodium Feta
- **Lunch**: Egg Salad on Whole Grain Toast
- **Dinner**: Cauliflower Rice with Tofu and Peas
- **Dessert**: Gluten-Free Blueberry Muffins
- **Snack**: Roasted Chickpeas with Paprika

Day 10

- **Breakfast**: Kale and Mushroom Omelette
- **Lunch**: Grilled Shrimp with Cilantro-Lime Quinoa
- **Dinner**: Turkey Meatballs with Zucchini Noodles
- **Dessert**: Lemon Coconut Macaroons
- **Snack**: Peach and Mint Salad

Day 11

- **Breakfast**: Almond Flour Pancakes with a Berry Compote
- **Lunch**: Rice and Apple Salad with Cinnamon
- **Dinner**: Roast Chicken with Carrots and Potatoes
- **Dessert**: Rice Pudding with Stevia and Cinnamon
- **Snack**: Low-Sodium Tuna with Cucumber Slices

Day 12

- **Breakfast**: Rice Pudding with Vanilla and Stevia
- **Lunch**: Grilled Chicken Salad with Olive Oil and Lemon
- **Dinner**: Baked Tofu with Steamed Broccoli and Brown Rice
- **Dessert**: Frozen Banana Bites with Dark Chocolate
- **Snack**: Carrot Sticks with Low-Sodium Hummus

Day 13

- **Breakfast**: Rice Cakes with Almond Butter and Apple Slices
- **Lunch**: Lentil Salad with Cherry Tomatoes and Parsley
- **Dinner**: Grilled Shrimp with Cilantro-Lime Quinoa
- **Dessert**: Baked Apples with Almond Stuffing
- **Snack**: Hard-Boiled Eggs with Fresh Herbs

Day 14

- **Breakfast**: Chia Seed Pudding with Almond Milk and Berries
- **Lunch**: Vegetable Soup (Low-Sodium)
- **Dinner**: Grilled Turkey Burgers with Sautéed Spinach
- **Dessert**: Berry Sorbet with a Touch of Lime
- **Snack**: Greek Yogurt with Berries and Chia Seeds

Day 15

- **Breakfast**: Whole Wheat Toast with Avocado and Egg
- **Lunch**: Stuffed Bell Peppers with Ground Turkey and Quinoa
- **Dinner**: Baked Lemon Herb Salmon with Roasted Asparagus
- **Dessert**: Banana-Free Chocolate Avocado Mousse
- **Snack**: Rice Cakes with Almond Butter and Cucumber

Day 16

- **Breakfast**: Low-Potassium Oatmeal with Blueberries
- **Lunch**: Grilled Chicken Salad with Olive Oil and Lemon
- **Dinner**: Baked Lemon Herb Salmon with Roasted Asparagus
- **Dessert**: Banana-Free Chocolate Avocado Mousse
- **Snack**: Carrot Sticks with Low-Sodium Hummus

Day 17

- **Breakfast**: Egg White Scramble with Spinach and Bell Peppers
- **Lunch**: Quinoa and Cucumber Salad with Greek Yogurt Dressing
- **Dinner**: Chicken Stir-Fry with Bell Peppers and Zucchini
- **Dessert**: Apple Crisp with Oats and Cinnamon
- **Snack**: Rice Cakes with Almond Butter and Cucumber

Day 18

- **Breakfast**: Chia Seed Pudding with Almond Milk and Berries
- **Lunch**: Vegetable Soup (Low-Sodium)
- **Dinner**: Grilled Turkey Burgers with Sautéed Spinach
- **Dessert**: Homemade Coconut Milk Popsicles
- **Snack**: Greek Yogurt with Berries and Chia Seeds

Day 19

- **Breakfast**: Whole Wheat Toast with Avocado and Egg
- **Lunch**: Lentil Salad with Cherry Tomatoes and Parsley
- **Dinner**: Quinoa-Stuffed Eggplant
- **Dessert**: Low-Sodium Almond Butter Cookies
- **Snack**: Homemade Veggie Chips with Sweet Potato and Zucchini

Day 20

- **Breakfast**: Apple Cinnamon Quinoa Porridge
- **Lunch**: Rice and Bean Bowl with Roasted Veggies
- **Dinner**: Baked Cod with Garlic and Roasted Brussels Sprouts
- **Dessert**: Berry Sorbet with a Touch of Lime
- **Snack**: Air-Fried Sweet Potato Fries

Day 21

- **Breakfast**: Coconut Yogurt Parfait with Low-Sodium Granola
- **Lunch**: Tuna Salad with Cabbage and Light Mayo
- **Dinner**: Low-Sodium Beef Stir Fry with Snow Peas
- **Dessert**: Chia Seed Pudding with Cacao and Almond Butter
- **Snack**: Cottage Cheese with Pineapple

Day 22

- **Breakfast**: Homemade Fruit Smoothie (Banana-Free)
- **Lunch**: Stuffed Bell Peppers with Ground Turkey and Quinoa
- **Dinner**: Chicken and Sweet Potato Mash
- **Dessert**: Carrot Cake Energy Balls
- **Snack**: Almonds and Fresh Strawberries

Day 23

- **Breakfast**: Baked Sweet Potato with Cinnamon and Walnuts
- **Lunch**: Chickpea and Spinach Stir Fry
- **Dinner**: Grilled Salmon with Steamed Broccoli and Brown Rice
- **Dessert**: Baked Pears with Cinnamon and Walnuts
- **Snack**: Apple Slices with Almond Butter

Day 24

- **Breakfast**: Zucchini Fritters with Low-Sodium Feta
- **Lunch**: Egg Salad on Whole Grain Toast
- **Dinner**: Cauliflower Rice with Tofu and Peas
- **Dessert**: Gluten-Free Blueberry Muffins
- **Snack**: Roasted Chickpeas with Paprika

Day 25

- **Breakfast**: Kale and Mushroom Omelette
- **Lunch**: Grilled Shrimp with Cilantro-Lime Quinoa
- **Dinner**: Turkey Meatballs with Zucchini Noodles
- **Dessert**: Lemon Coconut Macaroons
- **Snack**: Peach and Mint Salad

Day 26

- **Breakfast**: Almond Flour Pancakes with a Berry Compote
- **Lunch**: Rice and Apple Salad with Cinnamon
- **Dinner**: Roast Chicken with Carrots and Potatoes
- **Dessert**: Rice Pudding with Stevia and Cinnamon
- **Snack**: Low-Sodium Tuna with Cucumber Slices

Day 27

- **Breakfast**: Rice Pudding with Vanilla and Stevia
- **Lunch**: Grilled Chicken Salad with Olive Oil and Lemon
- **Dinner**: Baked Tofu with Steamed Broccoli and Brown Rice
- **Dessert**: Frozen Banana Bites with Dark Chocolate
- **Snack**: Carrot Sticks with Low-Sodium Hummus

Day 28

- **Breakfast**: Rice Cakes with Almond Butter and Apple Slices
- **Lunch**: Lentil Salad with Cherry Tomatoes and Parsley
- **Dinner**: Grilled Shrimp with Cilantro-Lime Quinoa
- **Dessert**: Baked Apples with Almond Stuffing
- **Snack**: Hard-Boiled Eggs with Fresh Herbs

Day 29

- **Breakfast**: Chia Seed Pudding with Almond Milk and Berries
- **Lunch**: Vegetable Soup (Low-Sodium)
- **Dinner**: Grilled Turkey Burgers with Sautéed Spinach
- **Dessert**: Berry Sorbet with a Touch of Lime
- **Snack**: Greek Yogurt with Berries and Chia Seeds

Day 30

- **Breakfast**: Whole Wheat Toast with Avocado and Egg
- **Lunch**: Stuffed Bell Peppers with Ground Turkey and Quinoa
- **Dinner**: Baked Lemon Herb Salmon with Roasted Asparagus
- **Dessert**: Banana-Free Chocolate Avocado Mousse
- **Snack**: Rice Cakes with Almond Butter and Cucumber

Day 31

- **Breakfast**: Low-Potassium Oatmeal with Blueberries
- **Lunch**: Grilled Chicken Salad with Olive Oil and Lemon
- **Dinner**: Baked Lemon Herb Salmon with Roasted Asparagus
- **Dessert**: Banana-Free Chocolate Avocado Mousse
- **Snack**: Carrot Sticks with Low-Sodium Hummus

Day 32

- **Breakfast**: Egg White Scramble with Spinach and Bell Peppers
- **Lunch**: Quinoa and Cucumber Salad with Greek Yogurt Dressing
- **Dinner**: Chicken Stir-Fry with Bell Peppers and Zucchini
- **Dessert**: Apple Crisp with Oats and Cinnamon
- **Snack**: Rice Cakes with Almond Butter and Cucumber

Day 33

- **Breakfast**: Chia Seed Pudding with Almond Milk and Berries
- **Lunch**: Vegetable Soup (Low-Sodium)
- **Dinner**: Grilled Turkey Burgers with Sautéed Spinach
- **Dessert**: Homemade Coconut Milk Popsicles
- **Snack**: Greek Yogurt with Berries and Chia Seeds

Day 34

- **Breakfast**: Whole Wheat Toast with Avocado and Egg
- **Lunch**: Lentil Salad with Cherry Tomatoes and Parsley
- **Dinner**: Quinoa-Stuffed Eggplant
- **Dessert**: Low-Sodium Almond Butter Cookies

- **Snack**: Homemade Veggie Chips with Sweet Potato and Zucchini

Day 35

- **Breakfast**: Apple Cinnamon Quinoa Porridge
- **Lunch**: Rice and Bean Bowl with Roasted Veggies
- **Dinner**: Baked Cod with Garlic and Roasted Brussels Sprouts
- **Dessert**: Berry Sorbet with a Touch of Lime
- **Snack**: Air-Fried Sweet Potato Fries

Day 36

- **Breakfast**: Coconut Yogurt Parfait with Low-Sodium Granola
- **Lunch**: Tuna Salad with Cabbage and Light Mayo
- **Dinner**: Low-Sodium Beef Stir Fry with Snow Peas
- **Dessert**: Chia Seed Pudding with Cacao and Almond Butter
- **Snack**: Cottage Cheese with Pineapple

Day 37

- **Breakfast**: Homemade Fruit Smoothie (Banana-Free)
- **Lunch**: Stuffed Bell Peppers with Ground Turkey and Quinoa
- **Dinner**: Chicken and Sweet Potato Mash
- **Dessert**: Carrot Cake Energy Balls
- **Snack**: Almonds and Fresh Strawberries

Day 38

- **Breakfast**: Baked Sweet Potato with Cinnamon and Walnuts
- **Lunch**: Chickpea and Spinach Stir Fry
- **Dinner**: Grilled Salmon with Steamed Broccoli and Brown Rice
- **Dessert**: Baked Pears with Cinnamon and Walnuts

- **Snack**: Apple Slices with Almond Butter

Day 39

- **Breakfast**: Zucchini Fritters with Low-Sodium Feta
- **Lunch**: Egg Salad on Whole Grain Toast
- **Dinner**: Cauliflower Rice with Tofu and Peas
- **Dessert**: Gluten-Free Blueberry Muffins
- **Snack**: Roasted Chickpeas with Paprika

Day 40

- **Breakfast**: Kale and Mushroom Omelette
- **Lunch**: Grilled Shrimp with Cilantro-Lime Quinoa
- **Dinner**: Turkey Meatballs with Zucchini Noodles
- **Dessert**: Lemon Coconut Macaroons
- **Snack**: Peach and Mint Salad

Day 41

- **Breakfast**: Almond Flour Pancakes with a Berry Compote
- **Lunch**: Rice and Apple Salad with Cinnamon
- **Dinner**: Roast Chicken with Carrots and Potatoes
- **Dessert**: Rice Pudding with Stevia and Cinnamon
- **Snack**: Low-Sodium Tuna with Cucumber Slices

Day 42

- **Breakfast**: Rice Pudding with Vanilla and Stevia
- **Lunch**: Grilled Chicken Salad with Olive Oil and Lemon
- **Dinner**: Baked Tofu with Steamed Broccoli and Brown Rice
- **Dessert**: Frozen Banana Bites with Dark Chocolate

- **Snack**: Carrot Sticks with Low-Sodium Hummus

Day 43

- **Breakfast**: Rice Cakes with Almond Butter and Apple Slices
- **Lunch**: Lentil Salad with Cherry Tomatoes and Parsley
- **Dinner**: Grilled Shrimp with Cilantro-Lime Quinoa
- **Dessert**: Baked Apples with Almond Stuffing
- **Snack**: Hard-Boiled Eggs with Fresh Herbs

Day 44

- **Breakfast**: Chia Seed Pudding with Almond Milk and Berries
- **Lunch**: Vegetable Soup (Low-Sodium)
- **Dinner**: Grilled Turkey Burgers with Sautéed Spinach
- **Dessert**: Berry Sorbet with a Touch of Lime
- **Snack**: Greek Yogurt with Berries and Chia Seeds

Day 45

- **Breakfast**: Whole Wheat Toast with Avocado and Egg
- **Lunch**: Stuffed Bell Peppers with Ground Turkey and Quinoa
- **Dinner**: Baked Lemon Herb Salmon with Roasted Asparagus
- **Dessert**: Banana-Free Chocolate Avocado Mousse
- **Snack**: Rice Cakes with Almond Butter and Cucumber

Day 46

- **Breakfast**: Low-Potassium Oatmeal with Blueberries
- **Lunch**: Grilled Chicken Salad with Olive Oil and Lemon
- **Dinner**: Baked Lemon Herb Salmon with Roasted Asparagus
- **Dessert**: Banana-Free Chocolate Avocado Mousse

- **Snack**: Carrot Sticks with Low-Sodium Hummus

Day 47

- **Breakfast**: Egg White Scramble with Spinach and Bell Peppers
- **Lunch**: Quinoa and Cucumber Salad with Greek Yogurt Dressing
- **Dinner**: Chicken Stir-Fry with Bell Peppers and Zucchini
- **Dessert**: Apple Crisp with Oats and Cinnamon
- **Snack**: Rice Cakes with Almond Butter and Cucumber

Day 48

- **Breakfast**: Chia Seed Pudding with Almond Milk and Berries
- **Lunch**: Vegetable Soup (Low-Sodium)
- **Dinner**: Grilled Turkey Burgers with Sautéed Spinach
- **Dessert**: Homemade Coconut Milk Popsicles
- **Snack**: Greek Yogurt with Berries and Chia Seeds

Day 49

- **Breakfast**: Whole Wheat Toast with Avocado and Egg
- **Lunch**: Lentil Salad with Cherry Tomatoes and Parsley
- **Dinner**: Quinoa-Stuffed Eggplant
- **Dessert**: Low-Sodium Almond Butter Cookies
- **Snack**: Homemade Veggie Chips with Sweet Potato and Zucchini

Day 50

- **Breakfast**: Apple Cinnamon Quinoa Porridge
- **Lunch**: Rice and Bean Bowl with Roasted Veggies
- **Dinner**: Baked Cod with Garlic and Roasted Brussels Sprouts
- **Dessert**: Berry Sorbet with a Touch of Lime

- **Snack**: Air-Fried Sweet Potato Fries

Day 51

- **Breakfast**: Coconut Yogurt Parfait with Low-Sodium Granola
- **Lunch**: Tuna Salad with Cabbage and Light Mayo
- **Dinner**: Low-Sodium Beef Stir Fry with Snow Peas
- **Dessert**: Chia Seed Pudding with Cacao and Almond Butter
- **Snack**: Cottage Cheese with Pineapple

Day 52

- **Breakfast**: Homemade Fruit Smoothie (Banana-Free)
- **Lunch**: Stuffed Bell Peppers with Ground Turkey and Quinoa
- **Dinner**: Chicken and Sweet Potato Mash
- **Dessert**: Carrot Cake Energy Balls
- **Snack**: Almonds and Fresh Strawberries

Day 53

- **Breakfast**: Baked Sweet Potato with Cinnamon and Walnuts
- **Lunch**: Chickpea and Spinach Stir Fry
- **Dinner**: Grilled Salmon with Steamed Broccoli and Brown Rice
- **Dessert**: Baked Pears with Cinnamon and Walnuts
- **Snack**: Apple Slices with Almond Butter

Day 54

- **Breakfast**: Zucchini Fritters with Low-Sodium Feta
- **Lunch**: Egg Salad on Whole Grain Toast
- **Dinner**: Cauliflower Rice with Tofu and Peas
- **Dessert**: Gluten-Free Blueberry Muffins

- **Snack**: Roasted Chickpeas with Paprika

Day 55

- **Breakfast**: Kale and Mushroom Omelette
- **Lunch**: Grilled Shrimp with Cilantro-Lime Quinoa
- **Dinner**: Turkey Meatballs with Zucchini Noodles
- **Dessert**: Lemon Coconut Macaroons
- **Snack**: Peach and Mint Salad

Day 56

- **Breakfast**: Almond Flour Pancakes with a Berry Compote
- **Lunch**: Rice and Apple Salad with Cinnamon
- **Dinner**: Roast Chicken with Carrots and Potatoes
- **Dessert**: Rice Pudding with Stevia and Cinnamon
- **Snack**: Low-Sodium Tuna with Cucumber Slices

Day 57

- **Breakfast**: Rice Pudding with Vanilla and Stevia
- **Lunch**: Grilled Chicken Salad with Olive Oil and Lemon
- **Dinner**: Baked Tofu with Steamed Broccoli and Brown Rice
- **Dessert**: Frozen Banana Bites with Dark Chocolate
- **Snack**: Carrot Sticks with Low-Sodium Hummus

Day 58

- **Breakfast**: Rice Cakes with Almond Butter and Apple Slices
- **Lunch**: Lentil Salad with Cherry Tomatoes and Parsley
- **Dinner**: Grilled Shrimp with Cilantro-Lime Quinoa
- **Dessert**: Baked Apples with Almond Stuffing

- **Snack**: Hard-Boiled Eggs with Fresh Herbs

Day 59

- **Breakfast**: Chia Seed Pudding with Almond Milk and Berries
- **Lunch**: Vegetable Soup (Low-Sodium)
- **Dinner**: Grilled Turkey Burgers with Sautéed Spinach
- **Dessert**: Berry Sorbet with a Touch of Lime
- **Snack**: Greek Yogurt with Berries and Chia Seeds

Day 60

- **Breakfast**: Whole Wheat Toast with Avocado and Egg
- **Lunch**: Stuffed Bell Peppers with Ground Turkey and Quinoa
- **Dinner**: Baked Lemon Herb Salmon with Roasted Asparagus
- **Dessert**: Banana-Free Chocolate Avocado Mousse
- **Snack**: Rice Cakes with Almond Butter and Cucumber

Conclusion

Living with kidney illness may seem daunting, particularly when you're initially diagnosed. The modifications to your food and lifestyle can feel like mountains too high to climb. But with each single step, you'll realize that regulating your kidney health is not only possible—it's powerful. It's about taking ownership of your health, making educated decisions, and adopting the lifestyle that enables you to flourish, not simply endure. By knowing what your body needs and how to nourish it correctly, you're not simply adding years to your life—you're boosting the quality of your existence.

Throughout this book, we've covered a number of kidney-friendly recipes, meal plans, and advice that can help you adapt to the dietary modifications essential for kidney health. But beyond the recipes and meals, this trip is about something far more significant: regaining control over your health. Yes, renal illness necessitates adjustments, but such changes don't have to be scary or disappointing. They may be an invitation to a new, more informed way of life, with meals that feed, invigorate, and support your body in the manner it requires.

The path to greater health starts with education. Knowing which meals are helpful and which ones to avoid is a critical aspect of the process. Every decision you make has an influence on how you feel, and being equipped with the correct tools, like the kidney-friendly foods and dietary advice in this book, makes all the difference. Managing renal illness is not about restriction; it's about finding innovative ways to enjoy a range of tasty, nutrient-rich meals that work for your body. It's about finding new foods, new recipes, and a fresh attitude to eating that promotes both your physical health and mental well-being.

As you continue this path, it's crucial to realize that perfection isn't the goal—progress is. There will be days when things don't go as planned, when you mess up, or when you feel upset. And that's alright. The trick is to keep focused on the greater picture, recognizing that each healthy decision you make is a success. Each meal that corresponds with your kidney-friendly requirements is a step forward, even if it's only one step at a time.

It's also crucial to give yourself grace throughout this process. Changing the way you eat, buying differently, cooking with new products, and adjusting to a new rhythm in the kitchen takes time. You may not always feel like you're getting things right, but that's part of the process. The most essential thing is that you're trying. Every effort you make—whether it's attempting a new dish, rearranging your kitchen to make healthier choices simpler, or experimenting with kidney-friendly snacks—adds up.

Remember that you're not alone in this path. Many individuals are living well with kidney disease, flourishing despite the hurdles, and they've learned to embrace their condition in ways that empower them. The goal is to surround oneself with support—whether that's via medical experts, support groups, or loved ones. Having a team behind you may make all the difference in your confidence and success. And that team may also include your kitchen: your pantry packed with kidney-friendly foods, your recipes that guide you, and your daily meals that feed you.

In the end, living well with kidney illness is all about empowerment. You are in charge. You have the capacity to make choices that promote your health, your lifestyle, and your long-term well-being. The road won't always be simple, but it's a one worth taking. And when you take it, you'll find more than just greater kidney function—you'll discover a new way of living, a new understanding for what your body requires, and a strong feeling of success as you continue to make the choices that will help you live your best life.

This book has given you the basis, but the next step is up to you. Your journey to empowerment is about taking what you've learned and applying it to your life in a manner that makes sense for you. Maybe it's picking a kidney-friendly breakfast that you adore. Maybe it's learning to read food labels more attentively, or dedicating up time for meal planning each week. Whatever it is, know that each step puts you closer to feeling your best and living a life that isn't defined by sickness, but by the choices you make to live well.

As you commence on this trip, be proud of the steps you're taking, no matter how tiny they appear. Your health, your choices, and your devotion are powerful. You have the capacity to live better, feel better, and prosper, even with kidney disease. So take a deep breath, believe in yourself, and go forth with confidence. Your best self is waiting.

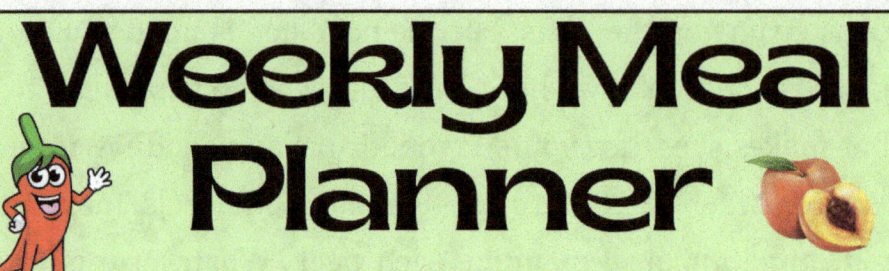

Weekly Meal Planner

	BREAKFAST	LUNCH	DINNER	SNACKS
MON				
TUE				
WED				
THU				
FRI				
SAT				
SUN				

GROCERY LIST

NOTES

www.ingramcontent.com/pod-product-compliance
Lightning Source LLC
Chambersburg PA
CBHW062328220526

45469CB00008B/2630